# Radiology

# RADIOLOGY

## *The Oral Boards Primer*

*By*

# AMIT MEHTA, MD

*South Texas Radiology Group, San Antonio, TX*

# DOUGLAS P. BEALL, MD

*Chief of Radiology Services, Clinical Radiology of Oklahoma
and Associate Professor of Orthopedic Surgery,
Oklahoma University Medical Center, Oklahoma City, OK*

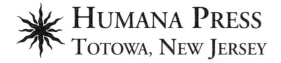

© 2006 Humana Press Inc.
999 Riverview Drive, Suite 208
Totowa, New Jersey 07512

**www.humanapress.com**

All rights reserved. No part of this book may be reproduced, stored in a retrieval system, or transmitted in any form or by any means, electronic, mechanical, photocopying, microfilming, recording, or otherwise without written permission from the Publisher.

The content and opinions expressed in this book are the sole work of the authors and editors, who have warranted due diligence in the creation and issuance of their work. The publisher, editors, and authors are not responsible for errors or omissions or for any consequences arising from the information or opinions presented in this book and make no warranty, express or implied, with respect to its contents.

Due diligence has been taken by the publishers, editors, and authors of this book to assure the accuracy of the information published and to describe generally accepted practices. The contributors herein have carefully checked to ensure that the drug selections and dosages set forth in this text are accurate and in accord with the standards accepted at the time of publication. Notwithstanding, since new research, changes in government regulations, and knowledge from clinical experience relating to drug therapy and drug reactions constantly occur, the reader is advised to check the product information provided by the manufacturer of each drug for any change in dosages or for additional warnings and contraindications. This is of utmost importance when the recommended drug herein is a new or infrequently used drug. It is the responsibility of the treating physician to determine dosages and treatment strategies for individual patients. Further, it is the responsibility of the health care provider to ascertain the Food and Drug Administration status of each drug or device used in their clinical practice. The publishers, editors, and authors are not responsible for errors or omissions or for any consequences from the application of the information presented in this book and make no warranty, express or implied, with respect to the contents in this publication.

This publication is printed on acid-free paper. ∞

ANSI Z39.48-1984 (American National Standards Institute) Permanence of Paper for Printed Library Materials.

Cover design by Patricia F. Cleary

Cover illustrations from Chapter 2, "Chest Radiology" and Chapter 9, "Pediatrics."

For additional copies, pricing for bulk purchases, and/or information about other Humana titles, contact Humana at the above address or at any of the following numbers: Tel.: 973-256-1699; Fax: 973-256-8341, E-mail: orders@humanapr.com; or visit our Website: www.humanapress.com.

**Photocopy Authorization Policy:**
Authorization to photocopy items for internal or personal use, or the internal or personal use of specific clients, is granted by Humana Press Inc., provided that the base fee of US $30.00 per copy is paid directly to the Copyright Clearance Center at 222 Rosewood Drive, Danvers, MA 01923. For those organizations that have been granted a photocopy license from the CCC, a separate system of payment has been arranged and is acceptable to Humana Press Inc. The fee code for users of the Transactional Reporting Service is: [1-58829-357-2/06 $30.00].

Printed in the United States of America. 10 9 8 7 6 5 4 3 2 1

eISBN: 1-59259-819-6

Library of Congress Cataloging-in-Publication Data

Mehta, Amit.
  Radiology : the oral boards primer / by Amit Mehta, Douglas P. Beall.
     p. ; cm.
  Includes bibliographical references and index.
  ISBN 1-58829-357-2 (alk. paper)
  1. Radiology, Medical--Examinations, questions, etc. 2. Oral examinations.
  [DNLM: 1. Radiology--United States--Examination Questions. WN 18.2 M498r 2006]
I. Beall, Douglas P. II. Title.
  R896.M44 2006
  616.07'572076--dc22
                                                                                    2006002111

# Preface

One of the most difficult and stressful times in the career of any diagnostic radiologist is in the preparation for the oral board exam given by the American Board of Radiology. Oral boards often engender more angst than the written boards because the potential questioning could include any possible question or combination of questions and because the exam requires physical participation.

*Radiology: The Oral Boards Primer* is designed to provide information that is typical of that found on the oral board examination for diagnostic radiology. Cases are provided to illustrate typical pathology and to provide a visual source for the construction of a differential diagnosis. Once the differential is mentally rendered, the mnemonics may be used as a memory aid and to augment any missing components of the differential that would be considered important. The chapters are organized as close to the oral boards exam format as possible. The cases should be examined, interpreted, and completed in a very rapid fashion, allowing for many cases to be reviewed in a single sitting. The vast majority of the cases contain prototypical representations of pathology allowing this text to be used as a memory aid and as a case reference source for many years after one has taken and passed the oral board examination.

The book can be used both during residency and at the time of review for the oral board examination. *Radiology: The Oral Boards Primer* will assist greatly in the preparation for this examination and will contribute to the assuredness and confidence that comes from being adequately prepared. As always, a text can only improve through evaluation and evolution, and we welcome your comments.

A CD-ROM edition of the book (ISBN 1-58829-928-7), sold separately, is available for use on the reader's PC or PDA.

***Amit Mehta**, MD*
***Douglas P. Beall**, MD*

# Acknowledgments

The following authors are acknowledged for their helpful contributions:

Yong C. Bradley, MD
Chief of Nuclear Medicine
Brooke Army Medical Center
San Antonio, TX

Nancy A. Brown, RT (R)(M)(M)(QM)
Radiologic Technologist
Wilford Hall Medical Center
San Antonio, TX

Liem Bui-Mansfield, MD
Chief of Musculoskeletal Radiology
Brooke Army Medical Center
San Antonio, TX

Neal Dalrymple, MD
Assistant Professor
Wilford Hall Medical Center
San Antonio, TX

David R. DeLone, MD
Wilford Hall Medical Center
San Antonio, TX

Judy Estroff, MD
Children's Hospital Boston
Boston, MA

Brian J. Fortman, MD
Assistant Professor
Medical University of South Carolina
Carolina Radiology Associates
Myrtle Beach, SC

Robert B. Good, MD
Chief of Interventional Radiology
Wilford Hall Medical Center
San Antonio, TX

David E. Grayson, MD
Assistant Professor
Wilford Hall Medical Center
San Antonio, TX

Lawrence Hofmann, MD
Assistant Professor of Radiology and Surgery
The Johns Hopkins Medical Institutions
Baltimore, MD

Melody E. Krumdieck, RT (R)(M)
Radiologic Technologist
Wilford Hall Medical Center
San Antonio, TX

Joe C. Leonard, MD
Professor of Radiology
University of Oklahoma Health Sciences Center
Oklahoma City, OK

Christopher J. Lisanti, MD
Chairman, Department of Radiology
Wilford Hall Medical Center
San Antonio, TX

John C. Morrison, MD
Division Chief, Nuclear Medicine
Wilford Hall Medical Center
San Antonio, TX

Fletcher M. Munter, MD
Chief of Neuroradiology
Brooke Army Medical Center
San Antonio, TX

Dan L. Nguyen, MD
Associate Professor of Radiology
Chief of Ultrasound
University of Oklahoma Health Sciences Center
Oklahoma City, OK

Jeffrey James Peterson, MD
Assistant Professor of Radiology
Mayo Clinic Jacksonville
Jacksonville, FL

David P. Raiken, MD
Division Chief, Abdominal Imaging
Wilford Hall Medical Center
San Antonio, TX

# Acknowledgments

Farid G. Ramji, MD, FRCPC
Assistant Professor of Radiology
Division of Pediatric Radiology
University of Oklahoma Health Sciences Center
Oklahoma City, OK

Todd S. Regier, MD
University of Oklahoma Health Sciences Center
Oklahoma City, OK

Randy Ray Richardson, MD
Wilford Hall Medical Center
San Antonio, TX

Richard Robertson, MD
Director of Neuroradiology
Children's Hospital Boston
Boston, MA

Thomas M. Seay, MD
Wilford Hall Medical Center
San Antonio, TX

Ernesto Torres, MD
Chief of Body Imaging
Brook Army Medical Center
San Antonio, TX

The following contributors were instrumental in gathering the images used throughout the volume:

Kevin P. Banks, MD
Department of Radiology
Wilford Hall Medical Center
San Antonio, TX

Scot E. Campbell, MD
Department of Radiology
Wilford Hall Medical Center
San Antonio, TX

Judy A. Estroff, MD
Associate Professor
Department of Radiology
Children's Hospital Boston
Boston, MA

Jason H. Eves, MD
Department of Radiology
Wilford Hall Medical Center
San Antonio, TX

Brian J. Fortman, MD,
Medical University of South Carolina
Carolina Radiology Associates
Myrtle Beach, SC

Chad W. Harston, MD
Department of Radiology
Wilford Hall Medical Center
San Antonio, TX

Todd M. Johnson, MD
Department of Radiology
Wilford Hall Medical Center
San Antonio, TX

Justin Q. Ly, MD
Department of Radiology
Wilford Hall Medical Center
San Antonio, TX

Victoria Trapanotto, DO
Department of Radiology
Children's Hospital Boston
Boston, MA

Eric E. Williamson, MD
Department of Radiology
The Mayo Clinic
Rochester, MN

# Contents

Preface ................................................................................................... v
Acknowledgments ............................................................................... vii
An Approach to the Oral Boards ...................................................... xiii

1. Musculoskeletal Radiology .............................................................. 1
2. Chest Radiology ............................................................................ 33
3. Gastrointestinal Radiology ............................................................ 59
4. Genitourinary Radiology ............................................................. 104
5. Head and Neck Radiology ........................................................... 135
6. Vascular and Interventional ......................................................... 161
7. Nuclear Medicine ........................................................................ 177
8. Ultrasound ................................................................................... 211
9. Pediatrics ..................................................................................... 303
10. Breast .......................................................................................... 333
11. Neuroradiology ........................................................................... 347

# An Approach to the Oral Boards

The oral boards attempt to cover a large amount of material in a short period of time. It is to your advantage to cover as much material as you can so that if one case does not go well, you have a big denominator to limit the significance of that particular case. As such, it is important to have an organized approach to each case. This not only shows the examiner that you are prepared, but also allows for an intelligent discussion.

## THE 5Ds

**Data**
**Detect**
**Describe**
**Differential**
**Diagnose**

For each case use this approach.

### 1. Data

This is a quick description of the study and any pertinent data the examiner gives you: "This is a contrast-enhanced computed tomography scan of the chest in a 42-yr-old African-American female with a 1-yr history of shortness of breath."

### 2. Detect

After a quick review of the image, show the examiner you have found the pertinent abnormality: "The abnormality is throughout both lungs radiating from the hilar regions along the bronchovascular bundles."

### 3. Describe

Take a brief moment to describe the abnormality to show the examiner you are focusing on the correct finding. If you have incorrectly detected or described the abnormality, the examiner will redirect you to the correct path: "There is soft tissue opacity that spreads along the bronchovascular bundles from both hila. There is associated lymphadenopathy in both hilar regions and the mediastinum."

### 4. Differential

Use the mnemonics in this text to give a quick differential diagnosis: My top four considerations for this constellation of findings would include the following:

Sarcoidosis
Histoplasmosis or TB
Amyloidosis
Metastasis

## 5. Diagnose

Of the differential diagnoses you have provided, give the examiner your top choice and a reason: "Of these differential diagnoses, my top choice is sarcoidosis. The combination of the patient's demographic data and the finding of spread along the bronchovascular bundles associated with lymphadenopathy best supports this diagnosis."

# 1
# Musculoskeletal Radiology

*Includes plain film diagnosis in all areas of the musculoskeletal system plus any related special or imaging procedures, including CT, interventional techniques, and MRI.*

## GENERAL CASE CATEGORIES
1. General including Metabolic
2. Congenital
3. Tumors
4. Arthritis

# General

## BASILAR INVAGINATION
### PF ROACH
**P**aget disease
**F**ibrous dysplasia
**R**ickets
**O**steogenesis imperfecta, Osteomalacia
**A**chondroplasia
**C**leidocranial dysplasia
**H**yperparathyroidism, Hurler syndrome

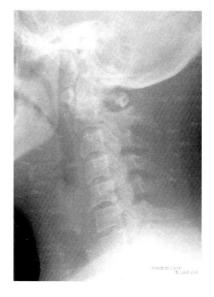

# SUBCHONDRAL CYSTS

## COORS

**C**PPD
**O**steoarthritis
**O**steonecrosis
**R**heumatoid arthritis
**S**ynovial-based tumors

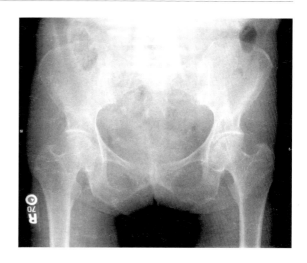

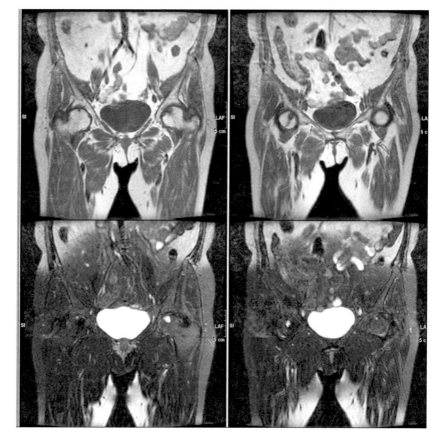

# ACETABULAR PROTRUSION

## PROTrusion

**P**aget disease
**R**heumatoid arthritis
**O**steomalacia
**T**rauma

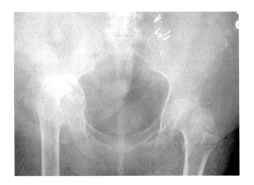

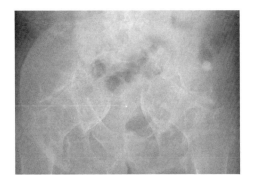

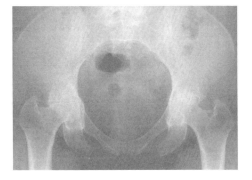

## STERNOCLAVICULAR SCLEROSIS
### STOP

**S**APHO syndrome
**T**raumatic osteolysis
**O**steomyelitis/Osteosarcoma
**P**agets

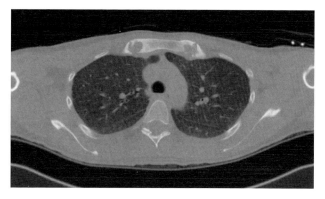

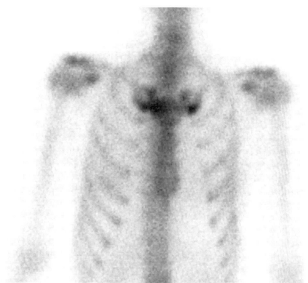

## DISTAL CLAVICLE EROSION
### SHIRT

**S**cleroderma
**H**yperparathyroidism
**I**nfection
**R**heumatoid arthritis
**T**raumatic osteolysis

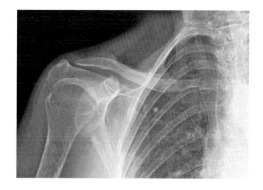

## SCLEROSIS-GENERALIZED

### R.S.M.O.P.M.M.P.F. (Regular sex mnemonic)

**R**enal osteodystrophy
**S**ickle cell disease
**M**yelofibrosis
**O**steopetrosis
**P**yknodysostosis
**M**astocytosis
**M**etastasis
**P**agets
**F**luorosis

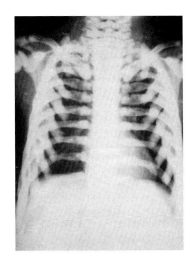

## OSTEONECROSIS

### ASEPTIC

**A**nemias
**S**ickle cell disease/SLE
**E**TOH/Exogenous steroids
**P**ancreatitis
**T**rauma
**I**nfection
**C**aisson's disease

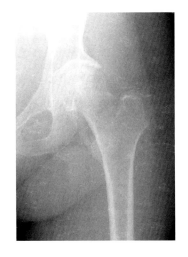

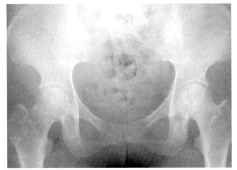

# ACRO-OSTEOLYSIS
## PINCH FO

**P**soriasis
**I**nfection
**N**europathic
**C**ollagen vascular disease
**H**yperparathyroidism
**F**amilial (Hadju Cheney)
**O**ther—polyvinyl alcohol

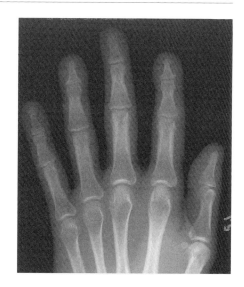

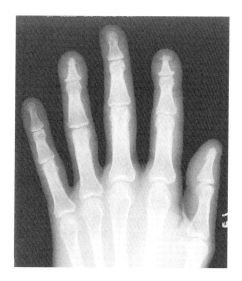

# CHONDRAL CALCIFICATION

## HOGWASH

**H**yperparathyroidism
**O**chronosis
**G**out
**W**ilson's Disease
**A**rthritis
**PS**eudogout
**H**emochromatosis

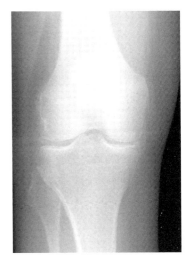

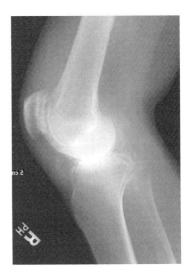

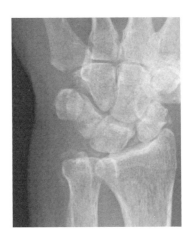

# Congenital

## ERLYMEYER FLASK

### CHONGO

Craniometaphyseal dysplasia
Hemoglobinopathies
Osteopetrosis
Niemenn Pick
Gaucher's Disease
Other

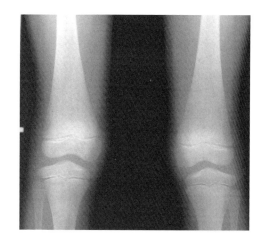

## METAPHYSEAL BANDS

### Dense

#### LINES

Lead poisoning
Infantile growth arrest
Normal, 3 yr
LEukemia treated
Syphillis

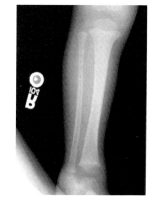

### Lucent

#### NORMAL TENDER LOVING CARE

Normal (neonates)
TORCH
Leukemia
Chronic illness

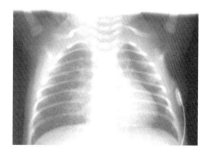

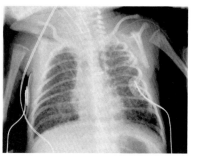

# GRACILE BONES

## NIMROD

**N**eurofibromatosis
**I**mmobilization
**M**uscular dystrophy
**R**heumatoid arthritis
**O**steogenesis imperfecta
**D**ysplasias

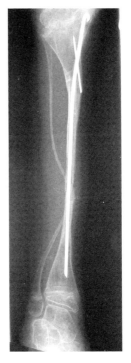
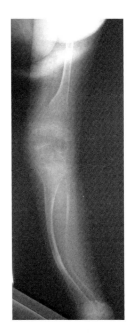
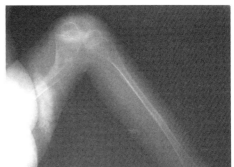
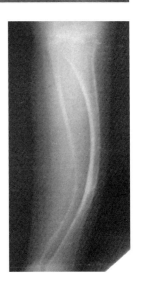

## MADELUNG DEFORMITY

### HITDOC

Hurler syndrome
Infection
Trauma
Dyschondrosteosis
Osteochondroma
Congenital–Turner's syndrome

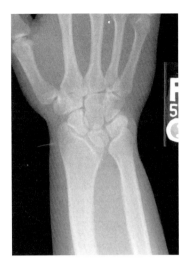

## SHORT METACARPALS

### BIC PEN

Basal Cell Nevus syndrome
Idiopathic
Chromosomal–Turner's syndrome
Pseudohypoparathyroidism/PseudoPseduo-
  hypoparathyroidism

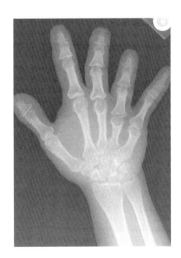

# Tumors

## DIAPHYSEAL LESIONS IN GENERAL
### CEMENT
Cysts
Enchondroma
Metastasis
Eosinophillic granuloma (EG)
Non-ossifying fibroma (NOF)
TB/infections

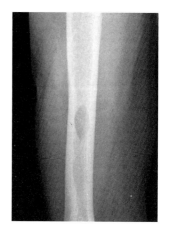

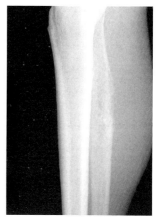

## CORTICAL LESION
### MOFOS
Metastasis
Osteomyelitis
Fibrosarcom
Osteoid osteoma
Stress fracture

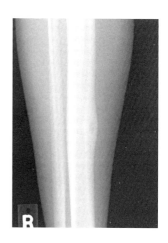

# Chapter 1 / Musculoskeletal Radiology

## ILIAC WING LESIONS
Fibrous dysplaisa
Unicameral bone cyst
Chondrosarcoma
Mets/Myeloma/Plasmacytoma
Ewings

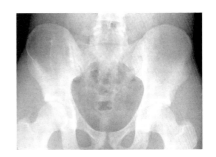

## VERTEBRA PLANA
### IMELT
Infection
Mets/Myeloma
EG
Lymphoma/Leukemia
Trauma

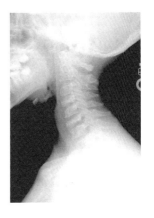

## BONY SEQUESTRUM
### LIFE
Lymphoma
Infection
Fibrosarcoma
EG

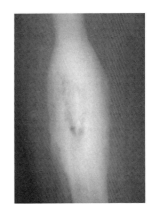

## RIB LESION
### FAME
Fibrous dysplasia
ABC
Metastatic/Myeloma/Lymphoma
EG/Enchondroma

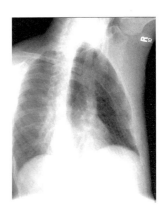

## EPIPHYSEAL LESIONS
### CIGS
Chondroblastoma
Infection
Giant cell tumor/Granuloma (EG)
Subchondral cyst

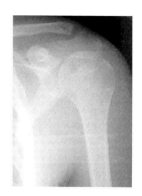

## FOCAL SCLEROTIC LESION
### HOME LIFE
Healed NOF
Osteoma
Metastasis
Ewing's sarcoma
Lymphoma
Infection/Infarct
Fibrous dysplasia
Enchondroma

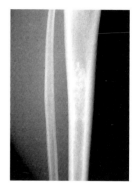

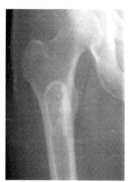

## PERMEATIVE LESIONS
### FIRE
Fibrosarcoma (Desmoid/MFH)
Infection
Round cell tumors
EG
Mets/Myeloma

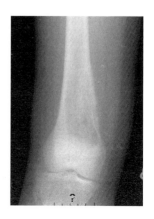

# SKULL LESION

## MEL TORME

Metastasis
EG
Lymphoma
TB
Osteomyelitis
Radiation
Mets
Epidermoid

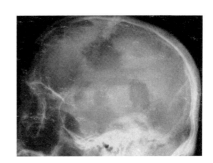

# TIBIAL LESION

## FOAM

Fibrous dysplasia
Osteofibrous dysplasia
Adamantinoma
Metastasis

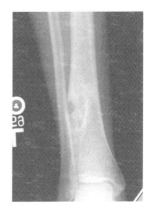

# POSTERIOR VERTEBRAL BODY LESION

## GO TAPE

Giant cell tumor
Osteoblastoma
TB
ABC
Paget disease
EG

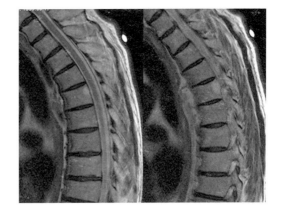

## CALCANEAL LESION
### BIG G

**B**one cyst-unicameral
**I**ntraosseous lipoma
**G**anglion
**G**iant cell tumor

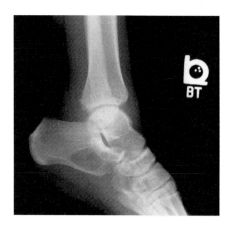

## FINGER TIP LESION
### GEMS

**G**lomus tumor
**E**pidermoid/Enchondroma
**M**etastasis (lung almost exclusively)
**S**arcoid

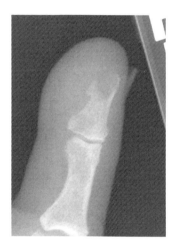

## SOFT TISSUE CALCIFICATION/OSSIFICATION
### My GHOSTS

**M**yositis ossificans
**G**out
**H**yperparathyroidism
**O**chronosis
**S**cleroderma/connective tissue disease
**T**umoral calcinosis
**S**arcoma (synovial cell)

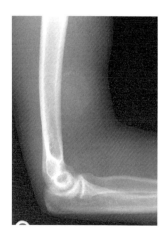

# Chapter 1 / Musculoskeletal Radiology

## SACRAL LESION

### CAN

Chondrosarcoma/Chordoma
ABC/GCT
Neurofibromatosis

And always Mets/Myeloma/Lymphoma

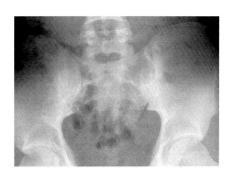

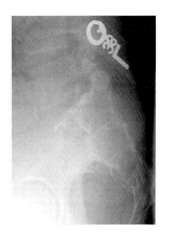

## FLUID-FLUID LEVEL

### HOT MASS

HemangiOma
Telangiectatic osteosarcoma
Metastasis
ABC/GCT
Synovial cell
Sarcoma

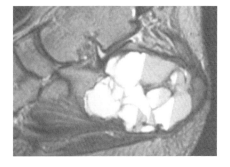

# Arthritis

## INFLAMMATORY ARTHRITIS

### 1. RF+

**Rheumatoid Arthritis**
–Symmetric

**SLE**
–Subluxation/nonerosive

**Scleroderma**
–DIP, PIP erosions
–Soft tissue $Ca^{2+}$
–Acroosteolysis

**Dermatomyositis**
–Soft tissue $Ca^{2+}$

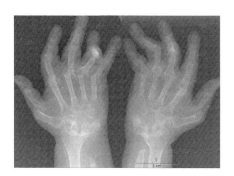

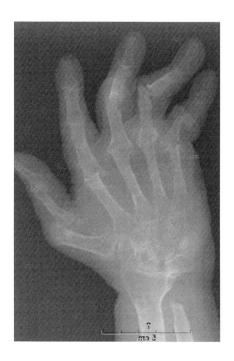

## 2. RF–

### Ankylosing Spondylitis
–SI joint involvement

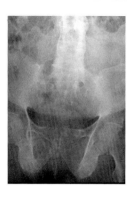

### Reiters
–Foot > Hand
–Bony Proliferation

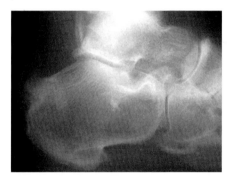 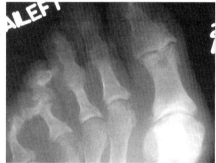

### Psoriasis
–Erosive
–Bony proliferation
–Asymmetric
–Sausage digit
–Ivory phalanx
–Pencil in cup

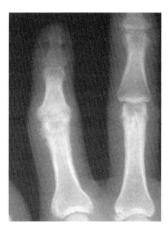 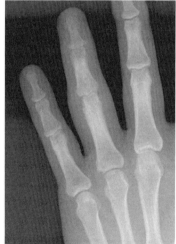

### Inflammatory Bowel Disease (IBD)
–Arthritis with IBD

## 3. EROSIVE OA

–Dip Joints

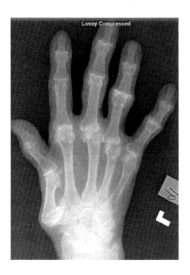

# CRYSTAL ARTHRITIS

## 1. DEPOSTION

### *Gout*
- Marginal erosions
- Overhanging edges
- Preserved joint space

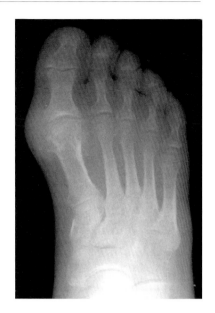

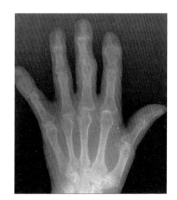

## CPPD
- ChondroCa$^{2+}$
- Cysts
- 2nd and 3rd MCP
- SLAC
- TFCCa$^{2+}$

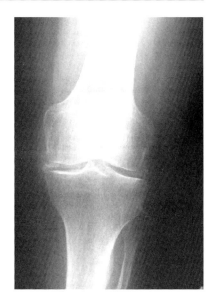

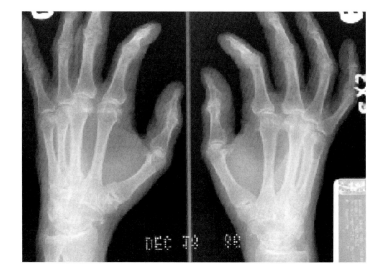

## 2. OTHER

### Hemochromatosis

### Acromegaly

### Other

Ochronosis
   –Disc calcification

Multicentric reticular histiocytosis
   –Symmetric
   –No osteopenia

Infection
   –Crosses Joint Space

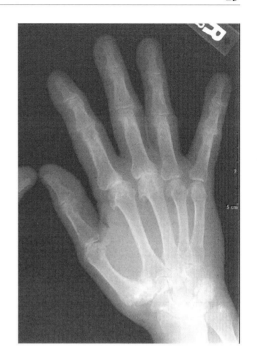

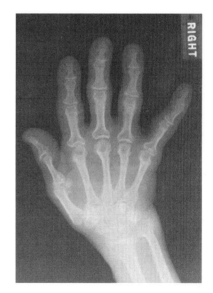

## OH MY GOD LESIONS

### VERY BIZARRE LOOKING GENERALIZED LESIONS THAT YOU HAVE NO IDEA WHAT IT IS, THINK OF:

Paget disease
Fibrous dysplasia
Neurofibromatosis
Charcot joints

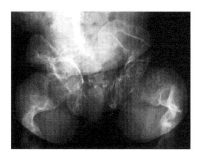

# Metabolic

## OSTEOPENIA

### GENERALIZED

Senile osteoporosis
Osteomalacia
Endocrine abnormalities
 –Cushings (too much)
 –Hypogonadism (too little)
Anemia/Myelofibrosis/Gauchers
 –Bone marrow
Congenital
 –Osteogenesis imperfecta
Hyperparathyroidism

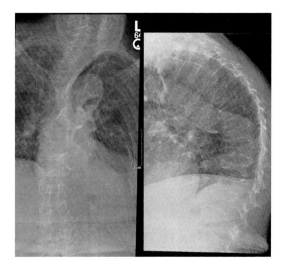
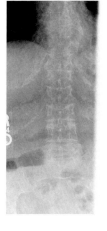
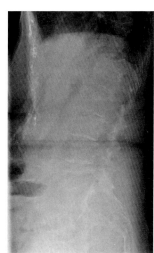

## FOCAL

Reflex sympathetic dystrophy (complex regional pain syndrome)
Disuse
Transient osteoporosis
Migratory osteoporosis

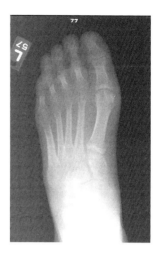

# SPINE

## CALCIFICATION OF THE ANNULUS FIBROSIS

Ankylosing spondylitis
  –Disks unremarkable
Ochronosis
  –Disks calcified
  –Abn SI joints

## OSTEOPHYTES

DISH
  –Disks unremarkable
  –Normal SI joints

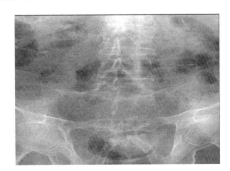

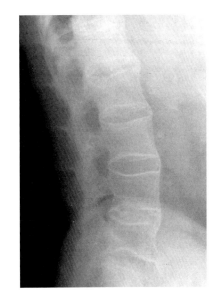

## SYNDESMOPHYTES

Psoriasis
Reiters

## MARGINAL OSTEOPHYTES

Spondylosis or degenerative

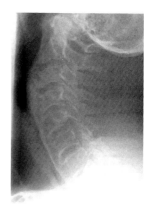

## OSTEOPHYTOSIS

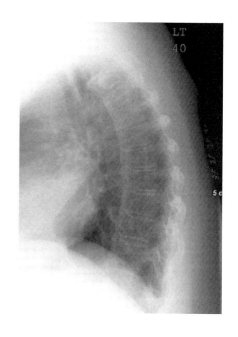

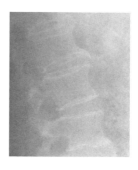
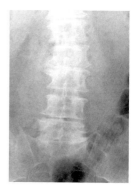

# ARTHRITIS BASICS AND ARTHRITIS BY LOCATION

**ABCDS**  
**A**lignment  
**B**one  
**C**artilage/calcifications  
**D**istribution  
**S**oft tissues

## *Wrist*

1st CMC, TFC—CPPD  
Radiocarpal joint—osteoarthritis  
CMC—gout (marginal erosions)

## *Hand*

### DIP + PIP

Osteoarthritis  
    –Osteophytes  
    –No erosions  
Erosive osteoarthritis  
    –Osteophytes  
    –Erosions  
    –Females  
Psoriasis/Reiters  
    –No osteophytes  
    –Erosions

### MCP + PIP

Rheumatoid  
    –Erosions  
    –No osteophytes  
    –Osteopenia  
Psoriasis/Reiters  
    –Erosion  
    –Bony proliferation

### MCP

Inflammatory  
    –Erosions  
CPPD/hemochromatosis  
    –Osteophytes

## *Foot*

### MTP JOINTS

RA  
Gout  
OA  
Neuropathic

### MIDDLE/HINDFOOT

RA  
Osteoarthritis

## *Hip*

### BONY PROLIFERATION

OA  
    –Superolateral migration  
Ankylosing spondylitis  
    –Axial migration  
    –SI joint involvement symmetric  
Psoriasis/Reiters  
    –Axial migration  
    –SI joint involvement asymmetric  
CPPD  
    –Chondrocalcinosis

### NO. PROLIFERATION

RA  
    –Acetabular protrusio  
    –Osteopenia

## Knee

**COMPLETE JOINT INVOLVEMENT**

RA
- No bony proliferation
- Osteopenia
- Cyst formation

JRA/hemophilia
- Wide femoral notch
- High density effusion

Psoriasis/Reiter's
- Asymmetric
- Bony proliferation

**MEDIAL INVOLVEMENT**

Osteoarthritis

**PATELLOFEMORAL INVOLVEMENT**

CPPD

## Shoulder

**GLENOHUMERAL JOINT**

CPPD
- vs osteoarthritis–not a weight-bearing joint

**ACROMIOCLAVICULAR JOINT**

Rotator cuff tear
- Glenohumeral joint spared

**TOTAL JOINT INVOLVEMENT**

Rheumatoid
- Symmetric

**NORMAL JOINT SPACE**

Hydroxyapatite crystal deposition disease

# NAMES TO KNOW

## UPPER EXTREMITY

| | LOCATION OF INJURY |
|---|---|
| Mallet Finger | Dorsal Base DP |
| Bennett's | 1st MC base, intraarticular |
| Rolando | Communited |
| Gamekeeper | 1st PP ulnar |
| Boxer's | 5th MC |
| Colle's | Distal radius |
| Smith's | Reverse colles |
| Chauffer's (Hutchinson's) | Radial styloid |
| Barton's | Dorsal rim |
| Rev. Barton's | Anterior rim |
| Nightstick | Ulnar shaft isolated |
| Monteggia | Ulna and radial + dislocation (elbow) |
| Galleazzi | Ulna and radial + dislocation (wrist) |
| Hill Sach's | Humeral head |
| Bankart | Glenoid |

## LOWER EXTREMITY

| | LOCATION OF INJURY |
|---|---|
| Jones | 5th MT base |
| Lisfranc | 2-5 MT |
| Choparts | Talonavicular and calcaneocuboid dislocation |
| Maisonneuve | Pronation external rotation injury- proximal fibula |
| Tillaux | Anterior tibial tubercle |
| Wagstaffe-Lefort | Fibular avulsion |

## SPINE

| | LOCATION OF INJURY |
|---|---|
| Jefferson | C1 lateral masses |
| Hangman | C2 pars Fx |
| Clay Shovelers | Posterior elements |
| Lefort I | Through maxilla |
| Lefort II | Nasal—inferior orbital rims |
| Lefort III | Nasal–orbits |

# 2
# Chest Radiology

*Includes plain film diagnosis, CT, MRI, and interventional techniques used in the diagnosis of diseases of the lungs, pleura, and mediastinum including the heart and great vessels.*

## LYMPHANGITIC CARCINOMATOSIS
### "CERTAIN CANCERS SPREAD BY PLUGGING THE LYMPHATICS"

**C**ervix
**C**olon
**S**tomach
**B**reast
**P**ancreas
**T**hyroid
**L**arynx

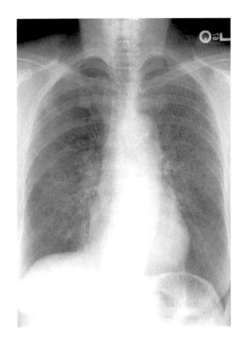

## BRONCHIOLITIS OBLITERANS

### CRITTERS

**C**OP/BOOP
**R**heumatoid
**I**nfectious-Swyer James
**T**ransplant
**T**oxins
**S**arcoid

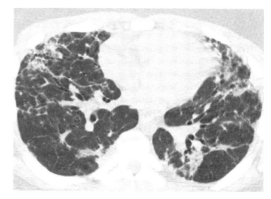

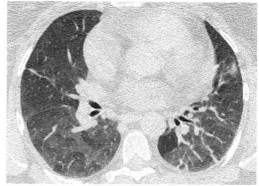

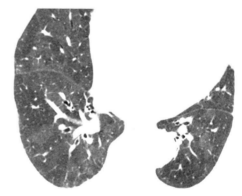

## MULTIPLE NODULES OR MASS >3 CM

### DAYS OF THE WEEK: MTWTFSS

**M**ets/Carcinoma/Lymphoma
**T**B/granuloma
**W**egeners
**R**heumatoid nodules/Round pneumonia
**F**ungal
**S**arcoid
**S**eptic pulmonary emboli

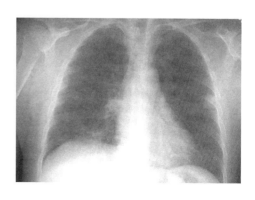

## COIN LESION <3 CM
### CHANGE

Carcinoma/Congenital
Hamartoma/Hematoma
AVM/Abscess
Neoplasm–mets
Granuoma
Esoteric-TB pneumonia

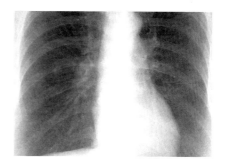
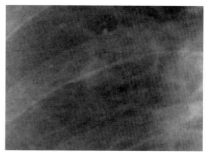
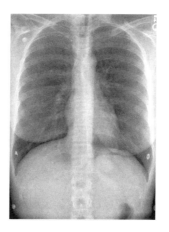
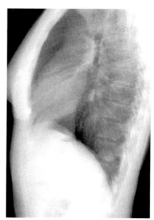
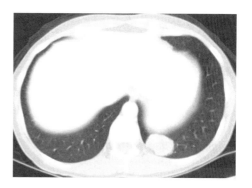

## A CT scan should be done to assess:

*Ca$^{2+}$ pattern*
   Benign: solid, lamellated, central
   Malignant: stippled, any other pattern.
   Density: fat - Hamartoma

*Margins:*
   Spiculated suggestive of carcinoma

*Enhancement*
   Four 1-min images >15HU suggestive

*Growth*

# CAVITY

## CAVITY

   **C**arcinoma-SCC
   **A**bscess-fungal/bacterial/TB
   **V**ascular-septic emboli
   **I**nflammatory-rheumatoid nodule
   **T**rauma-resolving contusion
   **Y**oung-bronchogenic cyst

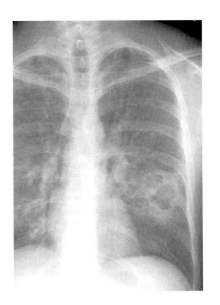

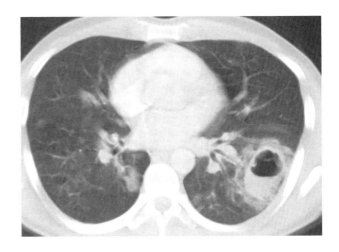

# CAVITY (*continued*)

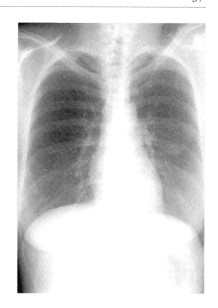

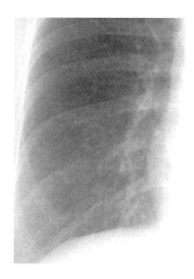

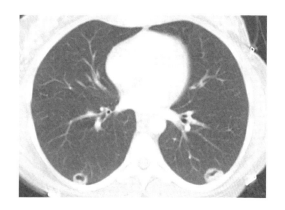

## BRONCHOVASCULAR SPREAD

### SKILL

Sarcoid
Kaposi
Infection–PCP/TB
Lymphoma
Lymphagitic spread

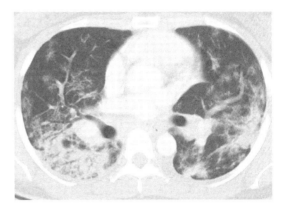

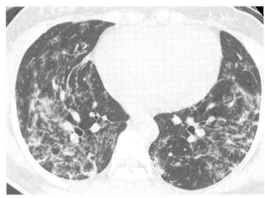

## UNILATERAL HYPERLUCENT LUNG

### POEMS

Poland syndrome/Pneumothorax
Oligemia/Obstruction (PE)
Emphysema
Mastectomy
Swyer James

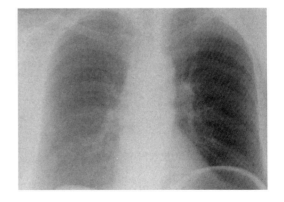

## ACUTE INTERSTITIAL DISEASE (RETICULAR)
### HELP

**H**ypersensitivity pneumonitis
**E**dema-Inhalation injuries
**L**ymphoproliferative
**P**neumonia-atypicals, PCP

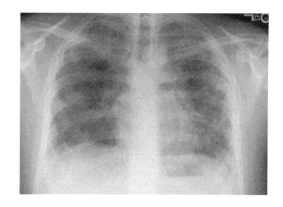

# CHRONIC INTERSTITIAL DISEASE (RETICULAR)
## PAGE CHUCK AT THE CIA RIGHT NOW, THERE'S DRUGS

### Upper Lung Zones
**P**neumoconiosis
**A**nkylosing spondylitis
**G**ranulomatous
**E**osinophillic
**S**arcoid/Silicosis

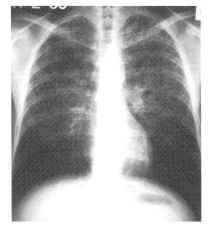

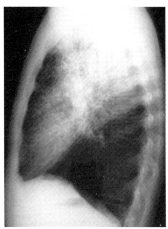

### Mid Lung Zones
Chronic **H**ypersensitivity

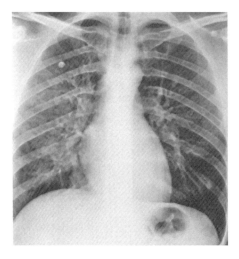
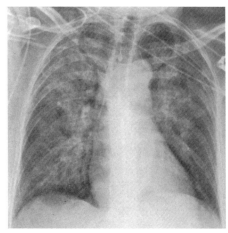

## LOWER LUNG ZONES

**C**ollagen vascular disease
**I**PF
**A**sbestos
**R**heumatoid
**N**F
**D**rug toxicity

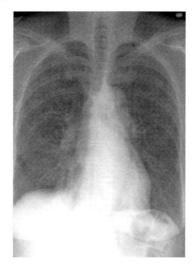
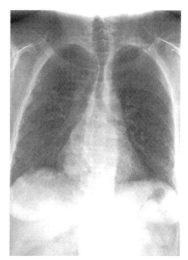
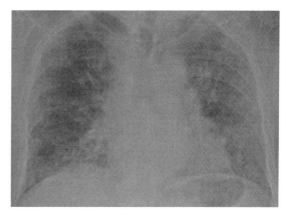
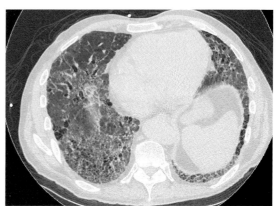

# ACUTE AIRSPACE DISEASE

## HELP LEGALIZE HEMP

### Diffuse

**H**emorrhage
**E**dema
**L**ymphoproliferative—esoteric
**P**neumonia

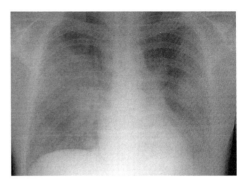

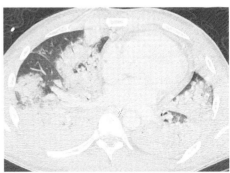

### Focal

**H**emorrhage-contusion/PE
**E**dema-inhalation (crack)
**M**I (RUL)
**P**neumonia

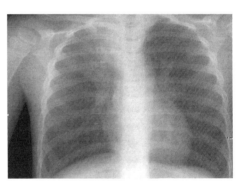

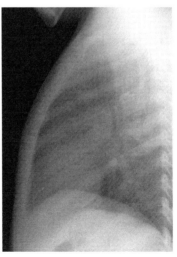

# CHRONIC AIRSPACE DISEASE

## PEBBLES

**P**AP/PCP/Pedema
**E**osinophillic pneumonia
**B**AC
**B**OOP
**L**ymphoma
**E**soteric-Wegener's/TB
**S**arcoid/Septic pulmonary emboli

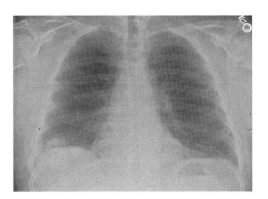

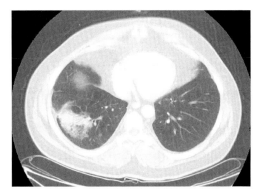

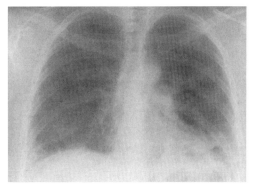

# GROUND GLASS DIFFUSE OPACITY

## SHAKE YOUR HIPS IN BED

Sarcoid
Hypersensitivity—smokers
Infection
Pneumonitis—DIP
Scleroderma/CVD
BOOP
Edema/aspiration
Drug toxicitiy

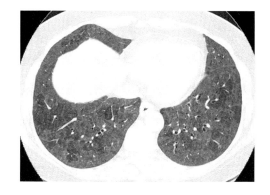

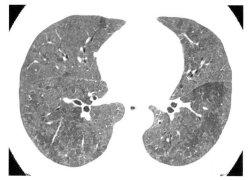

# CENTRAL OPACITIES EXTENDING FROM THE HILA OUTWARDS

## PPPP

PAP
Pulmonary edema
PCP
Pneumonia–atypical/influenza

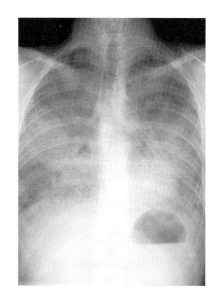

# MIDDLE MEDIASTINAL MASS

## HABIT

**H**ernia, Hematoma
**A**neurysm
**B**ronchogenic cyst/duplication cyst
**I**nflammation (sarcoidosis, histoplasmosis, coccidioidomycosis, primary TB in children)
**T**umors–remember the five Ls:
    Lung, especially oat cell
    Lymphoma
    Leukemia
    Leiomyoma
    Lymph node hyperplasia

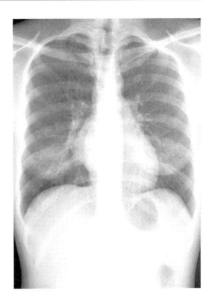

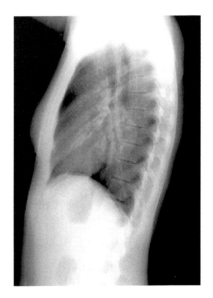

# RETICULAR (CXR)/CYSTIC OPACITIES (CT)

## ELECT CHIP

EG
LAM
Emphysema
CF
TS
Coccidiomycosis
Hydrocarbon
Infectious
PCP

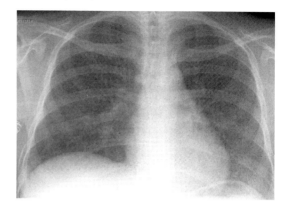

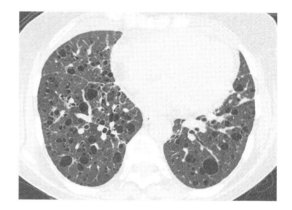

# FINGER IN GLOVE OPACITIES
## CACACA
CF
Asthma
Congential bronchial atresia
ABPA
Cancer
AVM

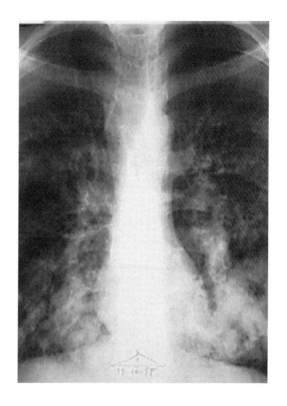

# CRAZY PAVING (CT)

## ACUTE
Edema
Hemorrhage

## CHRONIC
PAP
Sarcoid
PCP
Fibrosis

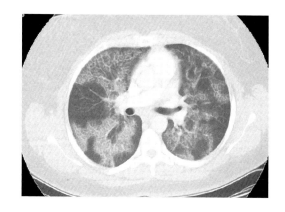

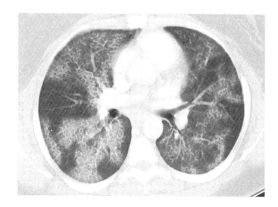

# END-STAGE LUNG (CXR)—ARCHITECTURAL DESTRUCTION

## TESSA

- **T**B
- **E**G
- **S**arcoid
- **S**ilicosis
- **A**RDS—The sequela of

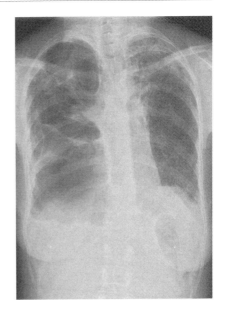

## CA$^{2+}$ NODULES

### MASH POX

Metastatic disease
Alveolar microlithiasis
Silicosis/siderosis
Histoplasmosis
Pox (Varicella)

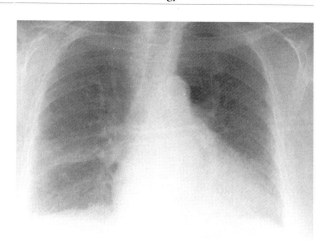

## TREE IN BUD OPACITIES (CT)

### MIT

Mucous plugging: Aspiration/Kartageners
Inflammatory plugging (PUS): TB/MAI
Tumor emboli (rare)

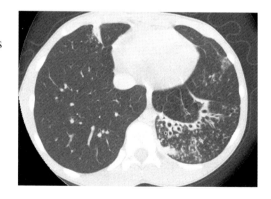

# NODULES (CT)

## DIFFUSE

### MISSLE

**M**ets
**I**nfection
**S**arcoid
**S**ilicosis
**L**ymphoma
**E**G

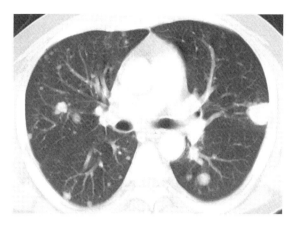

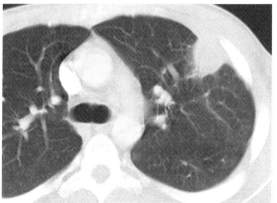

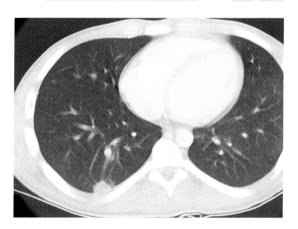

## PERILYMPHATIC

### A SKILL

Amyloid
Sarcoid
Kaposi's
Infection (PCP)
Lymphoma
Lymphang carcinomatosis

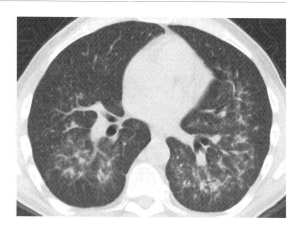

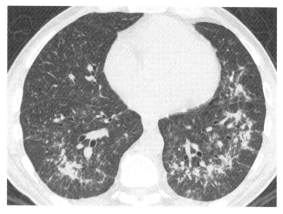

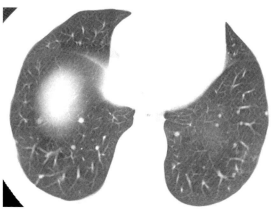

## CENTRILOBULAR

### HERB HAS GAS

Hypersen pneumonitis
EG
RB-ILD
BAC/BOOP
GVHD
VASculitis

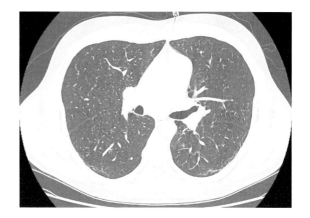

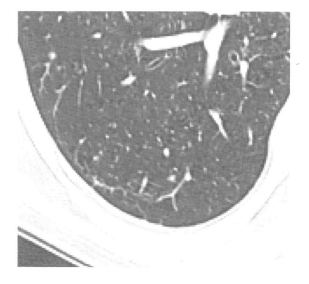

# BRONCHIECTASIS
## CAPT KANGAROO HAS MOUNIER KUHN

**C**ystic fibrosis
**A**BPA
**P**ostinfectious
**T**B
**K**artagener's
**M**ounier Kuhn

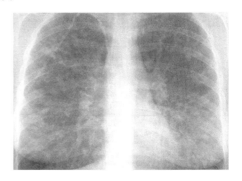

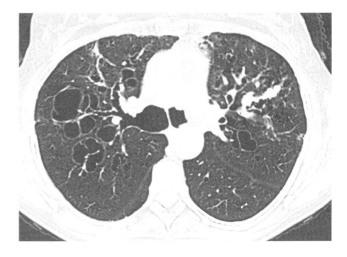

# TRACHEAL NEOPLASMS

## *Multiple*

### TRAM

**T**racheobronchopathia
**R**elapsing polychondritis
**M**etsastasis

## *Single*

### MATCH

**M**ucoepidermoid
**A**denoid cystic
**T**racheal SCC
**C**arcinoid
**H**amartoma

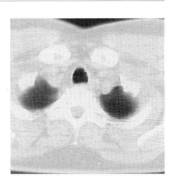

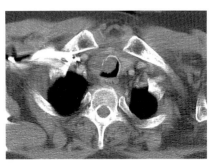

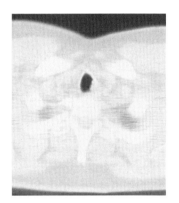

# Cardiac

## CARDIOMYOPATHY

### RESTRICTIVE

Sarcoid
Hemochromatosis
Amyloid
Endocardial fibroelastosis

### HYPERTROPHIC

Obstructive
Nonobstructive

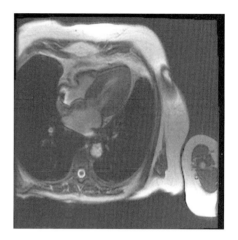

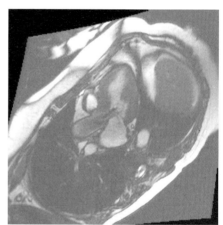

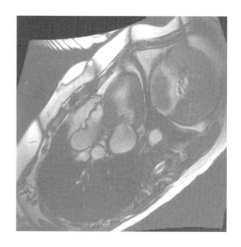

Dilated

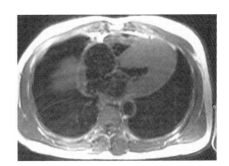

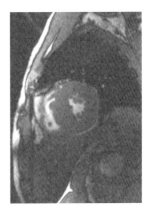

## PERICARDIUM

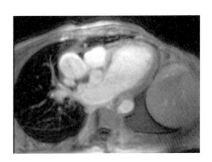

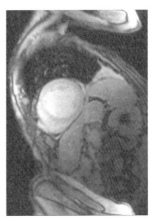

## $CA^{2+}$

Uremic
Viral
TB
Prior hemorrhage

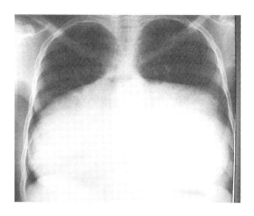

# 3
# Gastrointestinal Radiology

*Includes plain radiograph interpretation, contrast studies of the GI tract and abdominal imaging studies including CT, MRI, and ultrasound, plus interventional techniques related to the esophagus, stomach, small and large intestines, biliary tract, liver, spleen, pancreas, peritoneal cavity, and abdominal wall.*

## GENERAL

1. *The Gastrointestinal Mantra: Always consider the three following categories in the GI tract, almost all cases shown will encompass:*

    a. Neoplasm
    b. Infection
    c. Inflammatory

2. *In GI, when all else fails, think: TB, CROHN'S, LYMPHOMA, METS. It will save you 90% of the time.*

From: *Radiology: The Oral Boards Primer*
By: A. Mehta and D. P. Beall © Humana Press Inc., Totowa, NJ

## PLAIN FILM

*HAVE A SYSTEMATIC APPROACH ON THE BOARDS. It goes quickly so you must do this on all films.*

### "ABCD"

#### AIR (MISSING THESE = FAIL)
1. Portal vein
2. Emphysematous cholecystitis
3. Emphysematous pyelonephritis
4. Emphysematous cystitis
5. Retroperitoneal air
6. Free air
7. Pneumatosis

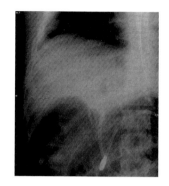

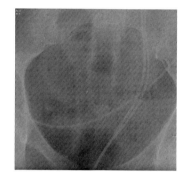

Chapter 3 / Gastrointestinal Radiology

# BOWEL
  Pattern
  Location
  Hernia

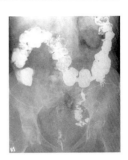

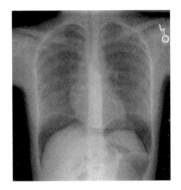

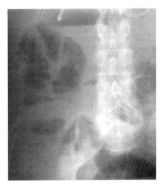

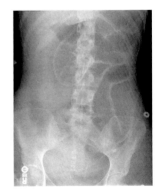

## Calcium

Gallbladder
Renal
Appendix
Bladder
Aneurysms

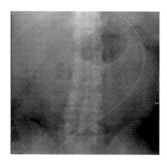
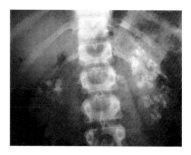
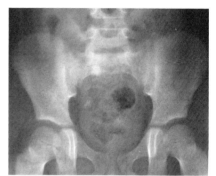
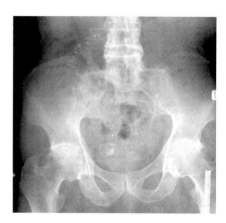
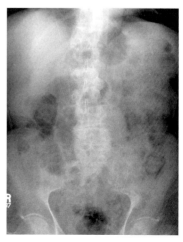

## DEM BONES

Lytic pedicles will signify RCC on board exams.

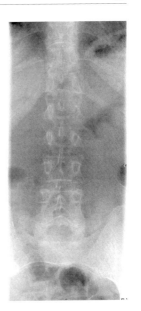

# ABNORMAL COLLECTION OF BARIUM ANYWHERE
## FED UP
- Fistula
- Extravasation
- Diverticulum
- Ulcer
- Perforation

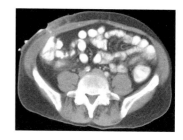
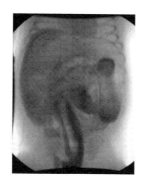
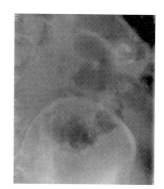
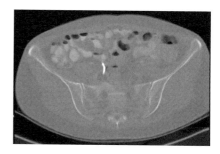
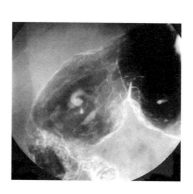
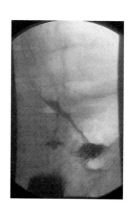

# Esophagus

## MASS

### CALL the MVP

Carcinoma
Adenoma/Polyp/Papilloma
Lymphoma
Leiomyoma
Metastasis
Varices
Papilloma

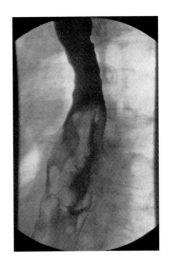

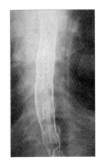

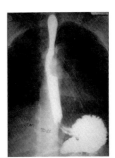

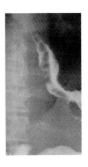

# ULCERATION/STRICTURE
## CAR RIMS
Caustic or NG/Crohn's
Adenocarcinoma
Reflux
Radiation
Infection/inflammatory
Metastasis
Skin – Bullous/Pemphigus

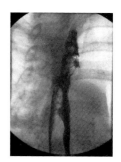

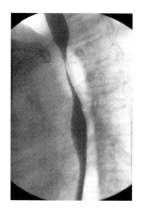

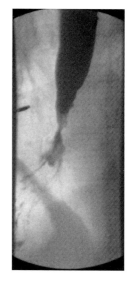

# ESOPHAGEAL FILLING DEFECTS

Candida
Glycogenic Acanthosis/Acanthosis Nigricans
Leukoplakia

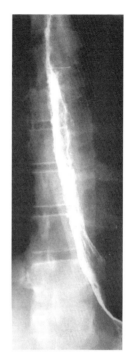

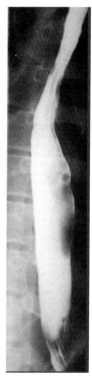

# ESOPHAGEAL MOTILITY DISORDER

## PRIMARY
Achalasia
Nonspec Esop Motility Dz
Presbyesophagus
DES

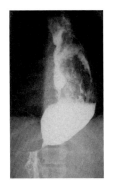

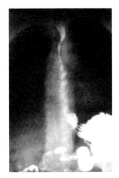

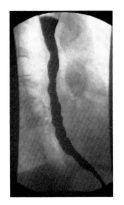

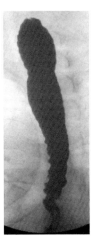

## SECONDARY

Scleroderma
Diabetes
Infection-Chagas
Esophagitis-reflux/radiation

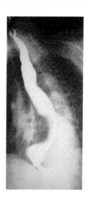

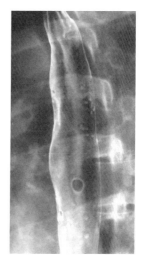

# DIVERTICULI

## High
PULSION-Zenker's

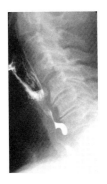

## Mid
TRACTION-TB/Histoplasmosis

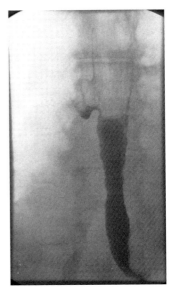

## Low
EPIPHRENIC

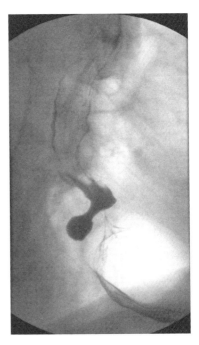

# Stomach

## GASTRITIS

Fold Thickening

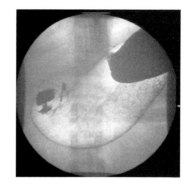
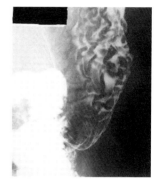

## GASTRIC ULCERS

### Benign

Thin folds
Beyond lumen
Eccentric crater
+ Hampton
N Peristalsis

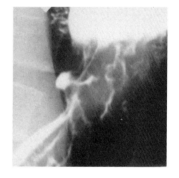

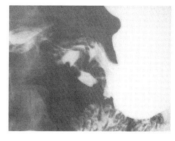

### Malignant

Thick fold
Within lumen
Central crater
− Hampton
Abn Peristalsis

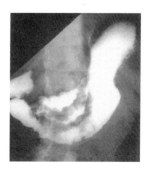

# APTHOUS ULCERS

## ACHE BABY

**A**SA/meds
**C**rohn's
**H**erpes
**E**TOH
**B**ehcet
**A**mebiasis
**B**ad AIDS
**Y**ersenia

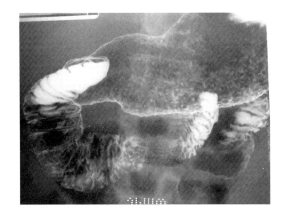

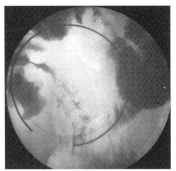

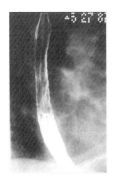

## ANTRAL NARROWING
### CTL SPINE (AS IN CTL: CERVICAL/THORACIC/LUMBAR)

Crohn's
TB
Lymphoma/carcinoma/mets

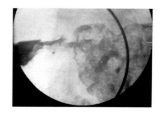

Sarcoid
Prior ulcer/Atrophic gastritis
Ingestion (caustic)
Eosinophic gastroenteritis

Chronic granulomatous dz childhood (Pediatrics only-for the 72)

## FOLD THICKENING
### LAMAZE CLASSES

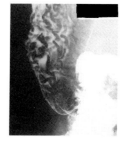

Lymphoma
Adenocarcinoma
Menetriers
Zollinger Ellison
Eosiniophillic gastritis

## GASTRIC MASS
### CALL ME

Carcinoma
Adenoma/Hyperplastic polyps
Lymphoma
Leiomyoma/Lipoma
MEtastasis

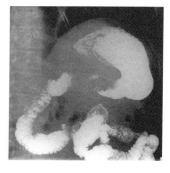

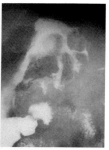

## CALL ME (continued)

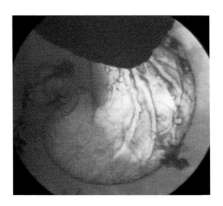

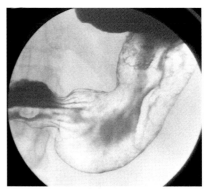

## LINITIS PLASTICA
### GRAM STAIN
> **G**ranulomatous infection (TB)/Crohn's/Lymphoma
> **R**adiation
> **A**denocarcinoma
> **M**etastasis-breast

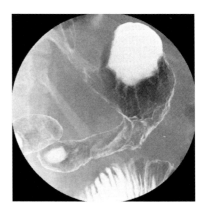

## BULLSEYE/TARGET LESION
### BLACK

**B**reast metastasis/Melanoma metastasis
**L**eiomyoma
**A**denocarcinoma
**C**ancer-lymphoma
**K**aposi

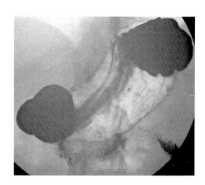

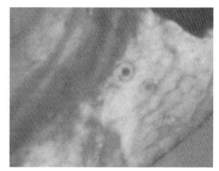

## DOUBLE CHANNEL PYLORUS
### ULCER

**U**lcer disease
**L**ymphoma
**C**rohn's
**E**ndoscopy induced injury
**R**adiation

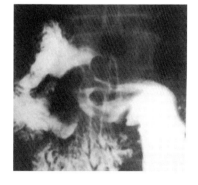

# Duodenum

## ANTRAL/DUODENAL FILLING DEFECTS

### BLED

Brunner's gland hyperplasia
Lymphoid hyperplasia
Ectopic gastric mucosa
Duodenitis

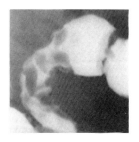

## BULBAR MASS

### ABCDE

**A**mpulla
**B**runner's gland adenoma
**C**rohn's
**D**uodenal adenocarcinoma
**E**ctopic pancreas

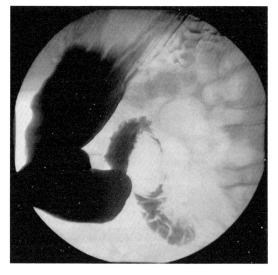

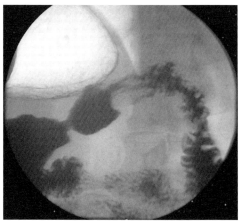

## DUODENAL ULCER
### PAT
Peptic ulcer
Adenocarcinoma
TB/Crohn's/Lymphoma

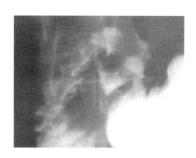

## DUODENAL FOLD THICKENING
### PAD LOCZS
**PA**ncreatitis
**D**uodenitis-ETOH/meds

**L**ymph**O**ma
**C**ystic Fibrosis/Crohn's
**Z**ollinger Ellison
**S**prue/strongyloides

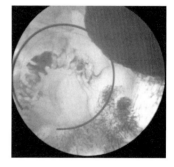

# Small Bowel

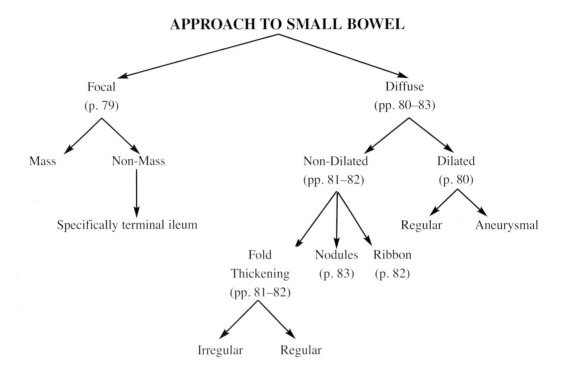

# FOCAL PROCESS

## ANYWHERE

Ischemia
Crohn's
Neoplasm
Radiation

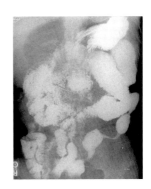

## *TERMINAL ILEUM (exclude appendix and cecal processes)*

TB
Crohn's
Lymphoma
Mets
Infection (specific to the TI)

### Your S Smells Totally Awful

**Y**ersinia
**S**higella
**S**almonella
**T**B
**A**ctinomycosis

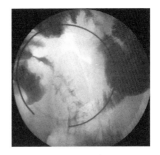

# DIFFUSE

## SMALL BOWEL

### Dilated

#### SOS

Sprue
Obstruction
Scleroderma

#### OR

| Wet Pattern | Dry Pattern |
|---|---|
| Sprue | Obstruction |
| Zollinger Ellison | Scleroderma |
| Lymphoma | Radiation |

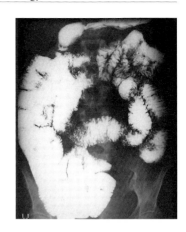

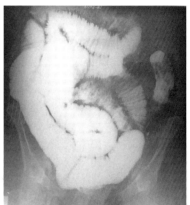

## SMALL BOWEL
### Aneurysmal Dilitation

#### MALL

Metastasis
Abscess/Hematoma
Lymphoma
Leiomyosarcoma

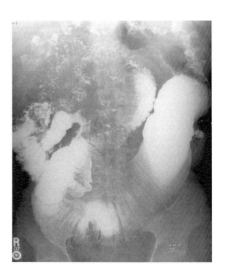

## SMALL BOWEL FOLDS

### Irregular Thickening

#### MALE COW

- **M**AI
- **A**myloid
- **L**ymphoma
- **E**osinophillic Gastroenteritis
- **C**rohn's
- **O**ther-Giardiasis
- **W**hipple

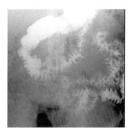

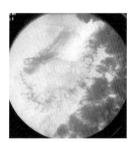

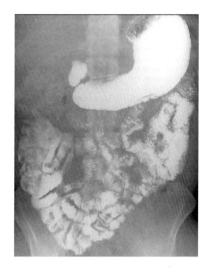

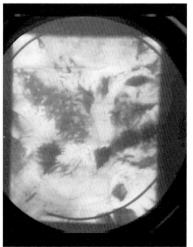

## SMALL BOWEL FOLDS

### Regular Thickened "Picket Fence"

**HEMORRHAGE**

HSP
Anticoagulation

**EDEMA**

CHF
Hypoproteinemia

**OTHER**

Lymphoma
Lymphagectasia
Radiation

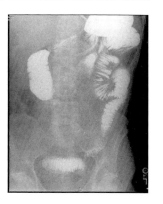

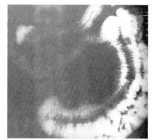

## SSMALL BOWEL

### Ribbon Bowel

#### A CUTE GIRL

**A**myloid
**C**ryptosporidiosis
**G**VHD
**I**schemia/Infection
**R**adiation
**L**ymphoma

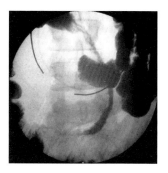

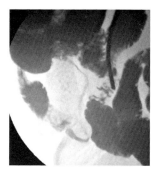

## SMALL BOWEL

### Masses

#### LACK

**L**eiomyoma
**A**denocarcinoma
**C**arcinoid
**K**aposi

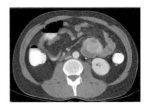

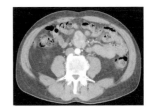

## SMALL BOWEL

### Nodules

#### MACE KILLS

**M**astocytosis/Macroglobunemia
**A**myloid
**C**rohn's
**E**osinophillic enteritis
**K**aposi

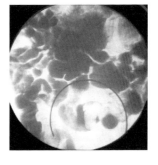

# Colon

## POLYPS

### SINGLE

Hamartomatous
Adenoma-tubular/tubulovillous/villous
Hyperplastic
Lymphoma
Inflammatory-UC/Crohn's

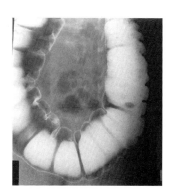

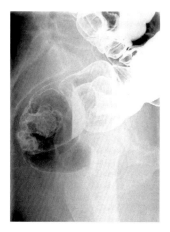

# MULTIPLE/POLYPOSIS

## 1. Hamartomas

Peutz-Jaeger: (MUCOCUTANEOUS)

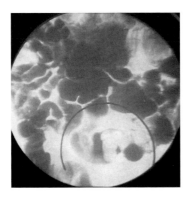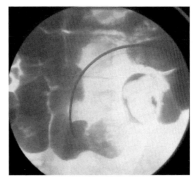

## 2. Hyperplastic

Juvenile Polyposis (Children are **HYPER**)

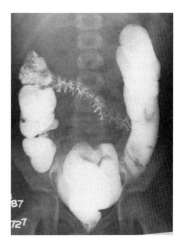

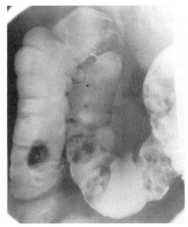

Cronkhite Canada:
  (CHECK STOMACH FOR POLYPS)

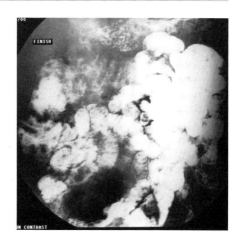

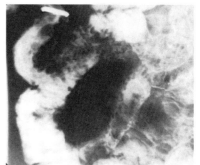

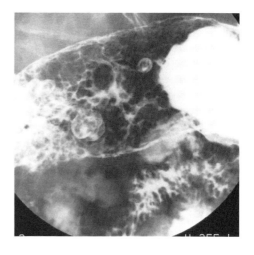

## 3. Adenomatous

### FiGhT

**F**amilial Polyposis

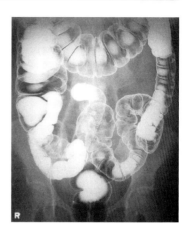

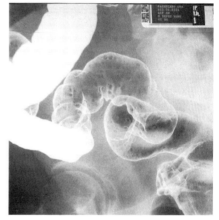

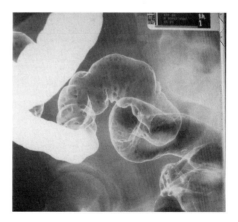

Gardner's

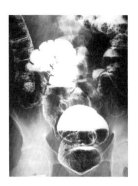
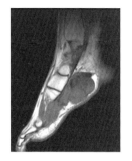
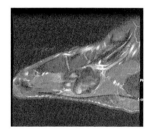
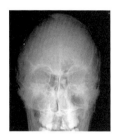
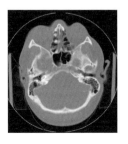
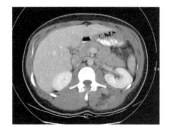

# Turcot

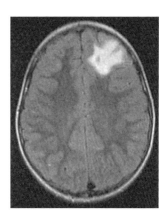
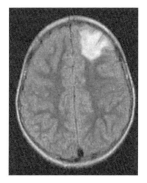
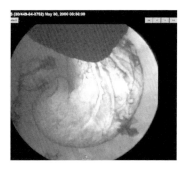
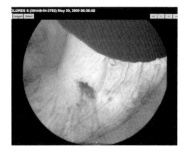

## SPICULATED SEROSA

### SEARS Credit Card

Serosal mets
Endometriosis
Abscess/Adhesion
Radiation
Swallowed foreign body

Crohn's
Carcinoid

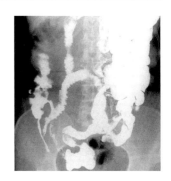

## PNEUMATOSIS

### CHIPS

COPD
Ischemia
Pneumatosis cystoides intestinalis
Scleroderma/Steroids

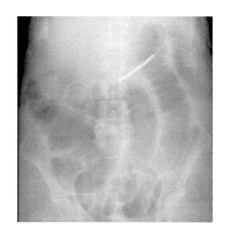

## SACCULATIONS

### MISC

Mets
Ischemia
Scleroderma
Crohn's

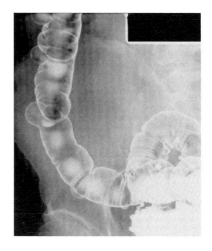

# BALD COLON

## I Use Radioactive LaxativeS

Ischemia
Ulcerative colitis
Radiation
Laxatives
Scleroderma

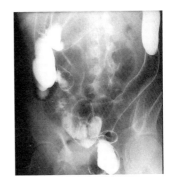

# GENERALIZED COLITIS

## I³NR

Infectious-E. coli/CMV
Inflammatory-Pseudom, Crohn's/UC
Ischemic -A. fib etc.
Neoplastic-lymphoma
Radiation

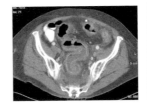 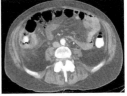

# FOCAL COLITIS

## CECUM-

### ABC

Amebiasis
Blastomycosis
CMV

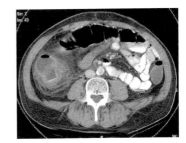

## RIGHT COLON-

Typhlitis, salmonella, shigella, TB, Diverticular bleed

## TRANSVERSE-

Pseudomembranous/CMV/E. coli
Pancreatitis/Stomach

## LEFT COLON-

Diverticulitis/CA
Ischemia at flexure
RCC

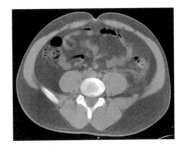

# APPENDIX

## INC

Infection
Neoplasm
  –Cystadenocarcinoma
  –Mucocele
Carcinoid

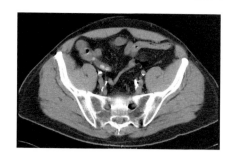

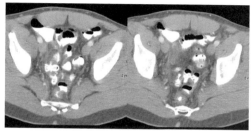

# RECTUM

## CLOGGED

Chlamydia
Lymphogranulomatous venerum
Gonococcus

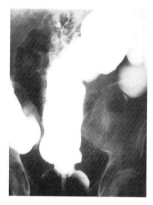

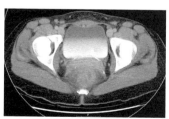

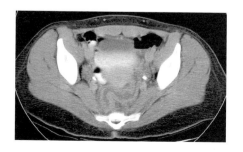

# Liver

## IN GENERAL:

1. Fatty or not? Always a favorite question

   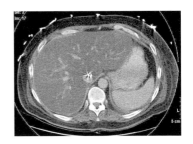

2. Cirrhotic or not? Makes one think of HCC every time

   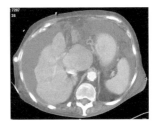

3. Portal vein—open or not? Consider HCC

   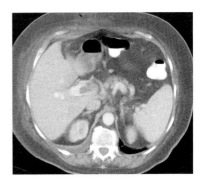

| DIFFUSE | FOCAL |
|---|---|
| ***Neoplasm***<br><br>• HCC<br>• Cholangiocarcinoma<br>• Lymphoma | ***Neoplasm***<br>**"LIVER CELL"**<br>• Benign<br>  – Adenoma<br>  – FNH<br>• Malignant<br>  – HCC<br>  – Fibrolamellar<br>  – Metastasis<br><br>**"BILE CELL"**<br>• Benign<br>  – Cystadenoma<br>• Malignant<br>  – Cystadenocarcinoma<br><br>**"MESENCHYMAL"**<br>• Benign<br>  – Hemangioma<br>• Malignant<br>  – Lymphoma |
| ***Infectious***<br>• Hepatitis | ***Infectious***<br>• Abscess |
| ***Inflammatory***<br>• Cirrhosis | |
| ***Other***<br>• Glycogen storage<br>• Hemochromatosis<br>• Fatty | |
| ***Vascular***<br>• Pre-Sinusoidal<br>  – Schistosomiasis<br>  – Cirrhosis<br>• Post Sinusoidal<br>  – Budd Chiari<br>  – CHF | |

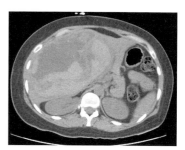

# Chapter 3 / Gastrointestinal Radiology

## IMAGES

*Diffuse Neoplasm HCC*

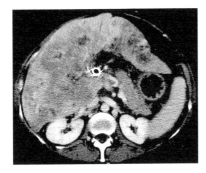
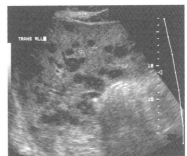

*Focal Neoplasm "Liver cell"*

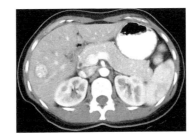
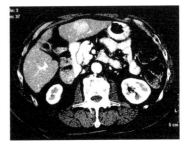

*Focal Neoplasm "Bile cell"*

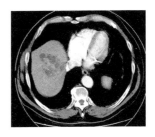

*Focal Neoplasm "Mesenchymal"*

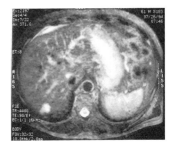

*Diffuse*
  *Infectious*

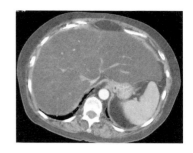

*Focal*
  *Infectious*

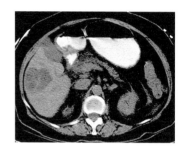

*Diffuse*
  *Inflammatory*

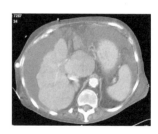

*Diffuse*
  *Other*

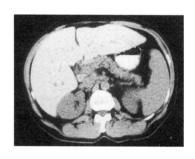

*Diffuse*
  *Vascular*

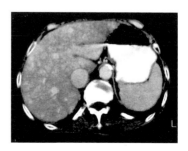

# BILE DUCT DILITATION

## High
HIV
PSC
Cholangiocarcinoma

## Confluence
Metastatic lymph nodes
Klatskin
HCC
GB

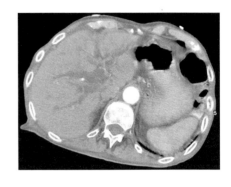

## Low
GB
Mirizzi
Post-instrumentation stricture
HCC

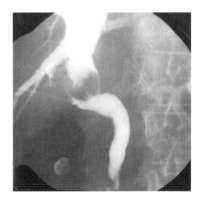

## Ampulla
Panc CA

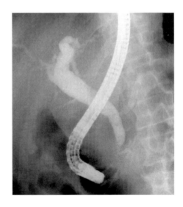

Stone

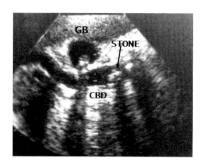

Cholangiocarcinoma

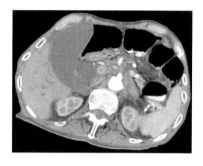

# BILE DUCT WALL THICKENING
## PAC-SAC

**P**ancreatitis
**A**scending cholangitis
**C**holangiocarcinoma
**S**clerosing cholangitis
**A**IDS cholangiopathy
**C**holedocholithiasis

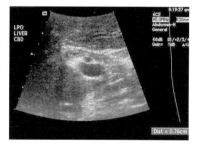

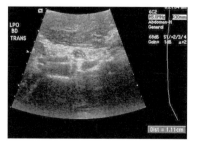

# Pancreas

## MASS

### *NEOPLASM*

#### *Gland*

##### AISLE

Adenocarcinoma
Islet
Solid and papillary epithelial neoplasm
Lymphoma
MEts

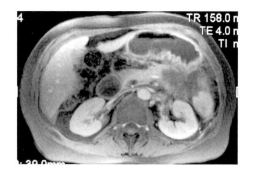

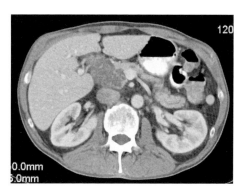

#### *Duct*

Macrocystic
Microcystic
IPMT (intraductal papillary mucinous
  tumor of the pancreas)

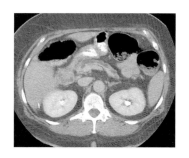

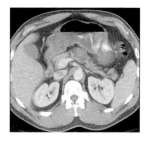

## Duct (continued)

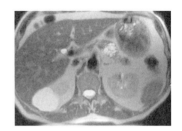

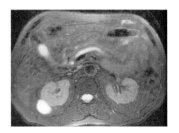

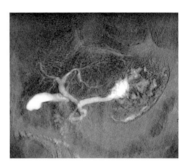

## INFLAMMATORY

### PANCREATITIS

Focal

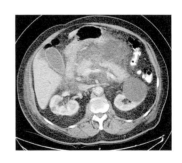

### OTHER

Abscess
Pseudocyst

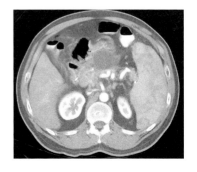

Real Cyst-VHL, PCKD

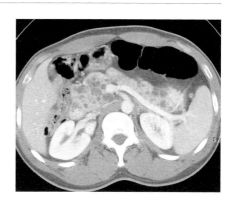

Choledochal cyst

# Spleen

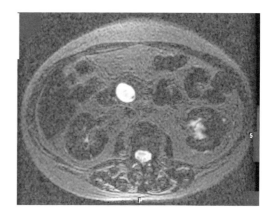

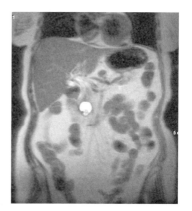

## CYSTIC LESION

### MATE

Metastasis
Abscess
Traumatic Cyst/Congenital Cyst
Echinococcal

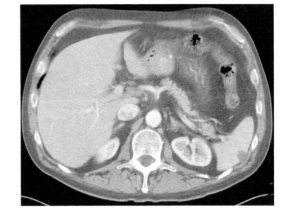

## SOLID LESION

Granulomatous disease
Metastasis: melanoma

Hemangioma/sarcoma
Infarct

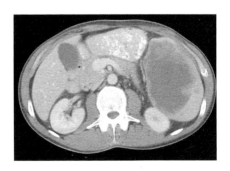

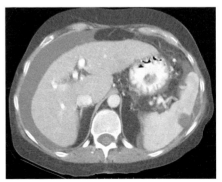

# Peritoneal Masses

### PEPPERCORN MELT

**P**eritoneal Carcinomatosis
**M**esothelioma
**L**ymphoma
**T**B

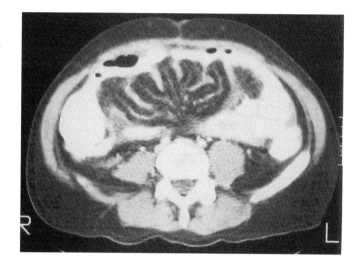

# 4
# Genitourinary Radiology

## NEPHROCALCINOSIS

### *Cortical*

#### COAGS

Cortical necrosis
Oxalosis
Alports
Glomerulonephritis
Sickle cell disease

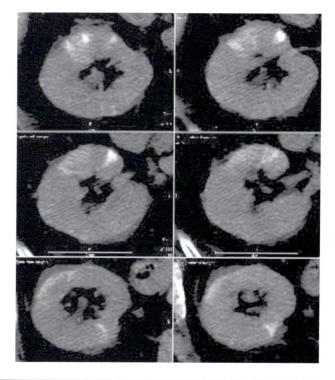

## Medullary

### MARCH

**M**edullary Sponge Kidney
**A**lkali
**R**TA
**C**ushing's syndrome
**H**PTH

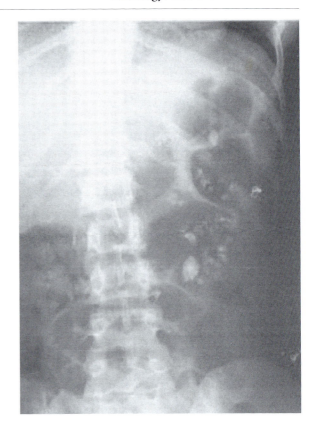

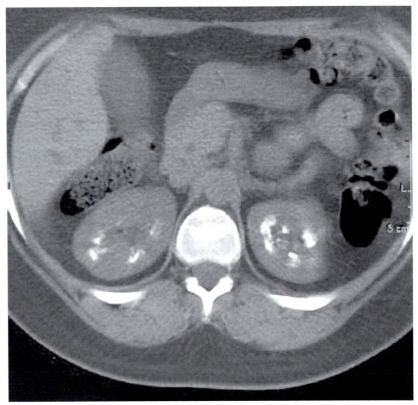

# PAPILLARY NECROSIS
## NSAID

**N**SAID
**S**ickle cell
**A**nalgesic
**I**nfection TB/Pyelo
**D**iabetes

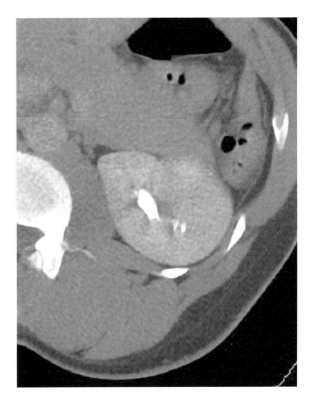

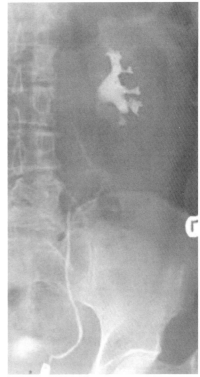

## NSAID (continued)

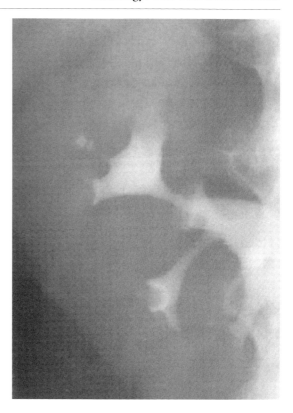

## BLADDER WALL CALCIFICATION

### STIR

**S**chisto
**T**b/TCC
**I**nterstitial
   or eosinophillic cystitis
**R**adiation

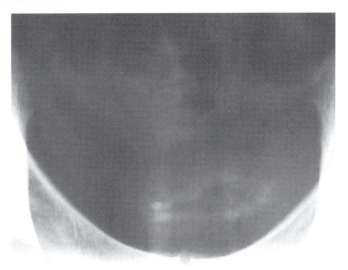

## URETERAL STRICTURE

### MISTER

**M**ets
**I**nflammation (stone)
**S**chisto
**T**b/TCC/Trauma
**E**ndometriosis
**R**adiation

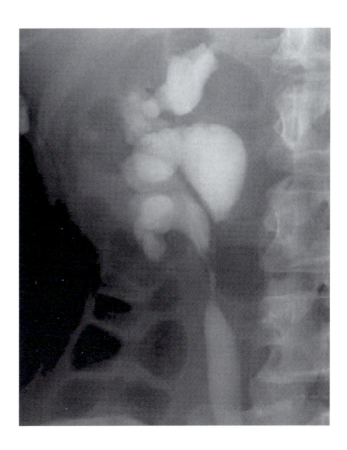

# URETERAL DEVIATION

## TAP YOUR FRIEND ON THE SHOULDER

### Lateral

#### TAP

Tumor (retroperitoneal)
Aneurysm/adenopathy
Peritonealization of ureters/post op

### Medial

#### FRIEND

Fibroid
RPF
Idiopathic
Enlarged prostate
Node dissection
Diverticulum

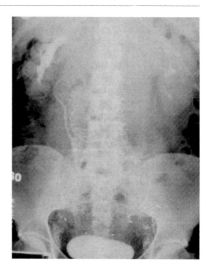
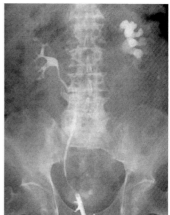
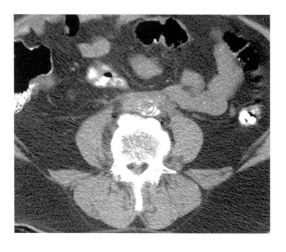
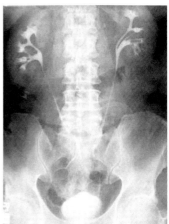

# RENAL MASS (CATEGORIZE BY ENTITY OR SHAPE)

## BY ENTITY

### *Tumor*

#### CYSTIC
Cystic RCC
MLCN
Mets

#### SOLID
Parenchymal—RCC
Mesenchymal—AML
Collecting System—TCC

#### OTHER
Mets
Lymphoma

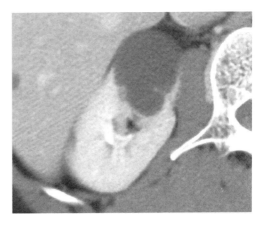

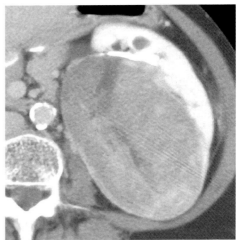

## Infection
Abscess
Pyelonephritis
XGP focal or diffuse

## Vascular
AVM
Hematoma

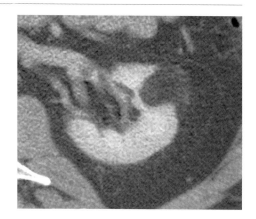
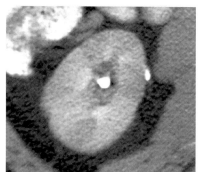
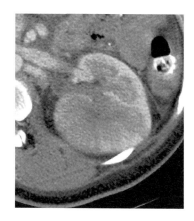
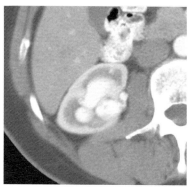

Chapter 4 / Genitourinary Radiology

## BY SHAPE

### Bean-shaped (entire kidney)
Metastasis
Diffuse RCC or TCC
Lymphoma
Infarction

### Ball-shaped (single mass)
RCC
TCC
Metastasis
Infection

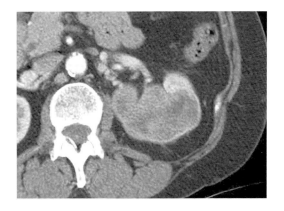

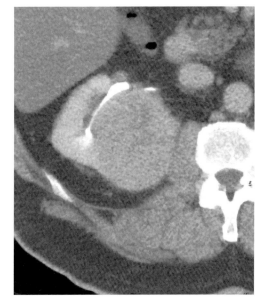

# WHEN DO YOU BIOPSY?

## When it changes management
- ? Metastatic disease
- ? Lymphoma (medical vs sx treatment)
  Single kidney
- ? Abscess

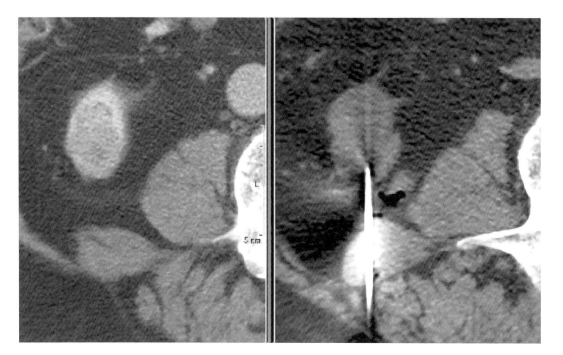

# INFUNDIBULAR NARROWING

| | | |
|---|---|---|
| Inflammatory | — | Stone |
| Infection | — | TB—"Phantom calyx" |
| Instrumentation | — | Trauma |
| TCC | — | "Oncocalyx" |

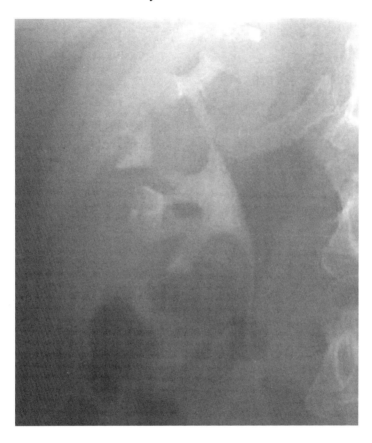

## URETERAL DILATATION

### PRESSURE OVERLOAD
Obstruction

### VOLUME OVERLOAD
Reflux
Diuresis

### INTRINSIC ABNORMALITY
Eagle Barrett
1° Megaureter

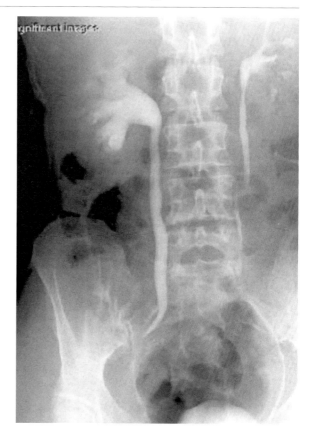

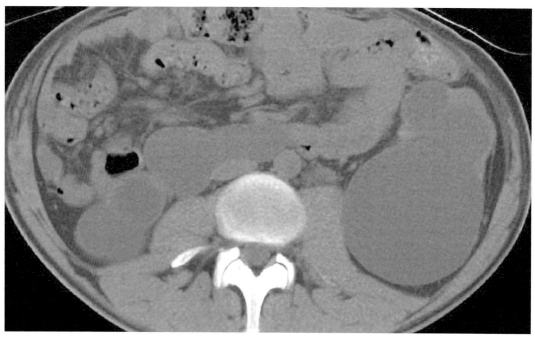

# DELAYED NEPHROGRAM

## PRERENAL

Hypotension
RAS

## RENAL

Glomerulonephritis
ATN
Papillary necrosis

## POSTRENAL

Crystals/proteins
Obstruction—ureteral or venous

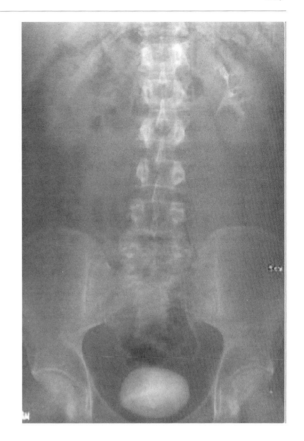

# STRIATED NEPHROGRAM

## MOP

**M**edullary sponge
**O**bstruction—vascular or ureteral (stone)
**P**yelonephritis

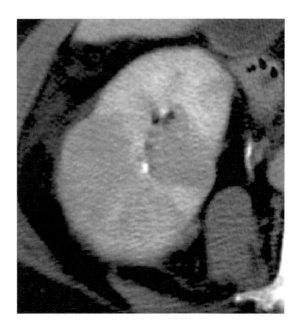

# RIM SIGN

## RAM

**R**enal vein thrombosis
**A**TN
**M**ain renal artery thrombus/avulsion

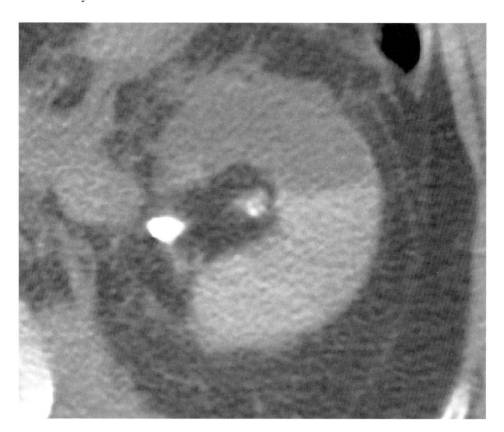

# UNILATERAL SMALL KIDNEY

Renal artery stenosis
Reflux nephropathy
Nephritis (chronic)
Congenital

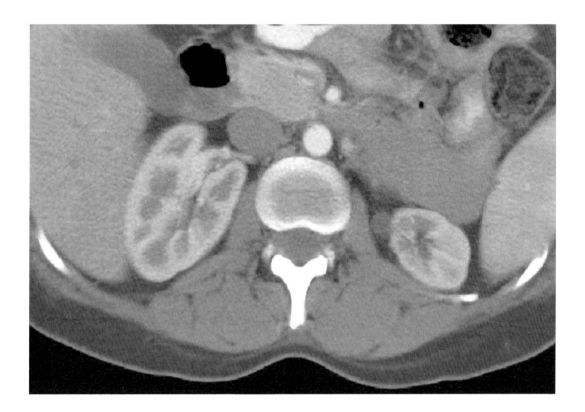

## RENAL AND URETERAL STONES
*(Radio-opaque + / Radiolucent −)*

|                 | Plain film | CT |
|-----------------|------------|----|
| Calcium oxalate | +          | +  |
| SMUX            |            |    |
|   Struvite |       |    |
|   Matrix   | −     | +  |
|   Uric acid |      |    |
|   Xanthine |      |    |
| Indinavir       | −          | −  |

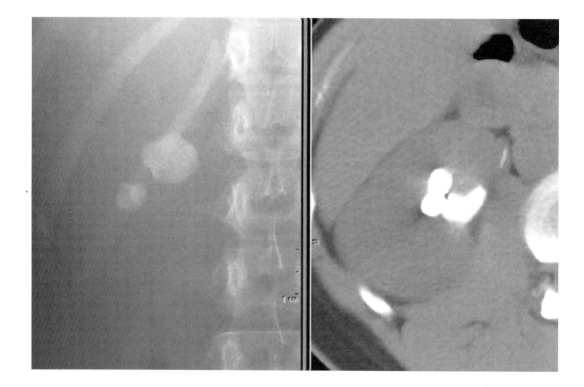

# Chapter 4 / Genitourinary Radiology

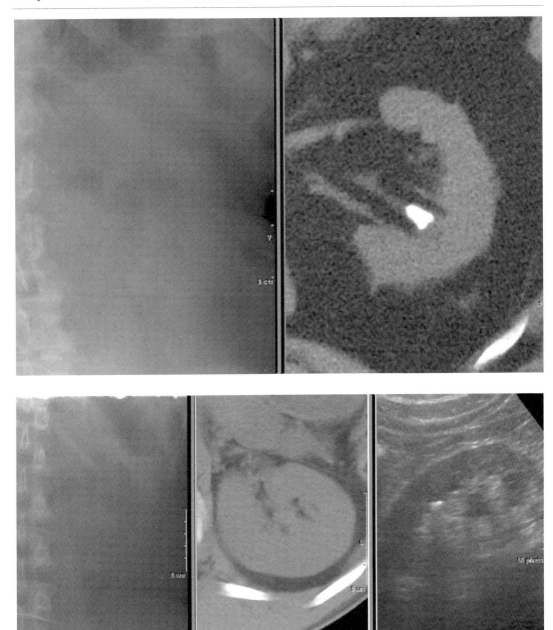

# RENAL TRANSPLANT

|  | Flow | FCN |
|---|---|---|
| ATN | Normal | Decreased <24 h |
| Rejection | Decreased | Decreased |
| Cyclosporine | Normal | Decreased >24 h |

# URETERAL FILLING DEFECTS

## Single

### 5CS

Calcium (stones)
Cancer (TCC)
Clots (blood)
Candida (fungus ball)
Crazy papilla (papillary necrosis)

## Multiple

### SLUMM

Stones
Leukoplakia
Ureteritis cystica
Malakoplakia
Metastasis—Melanoma

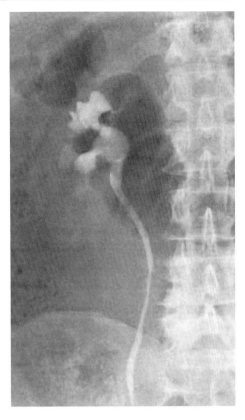

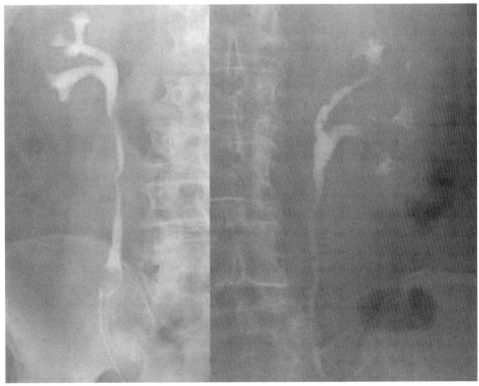

# PEAR-SHAPED BLADDER
## LAUNCH

**L**ipomatosis
**A**denopathy/lymphoma
**U**rinoma
**N**eurofibromatosis
**C**aval obstruction (collaterals)
**H**ematoma (trauma)

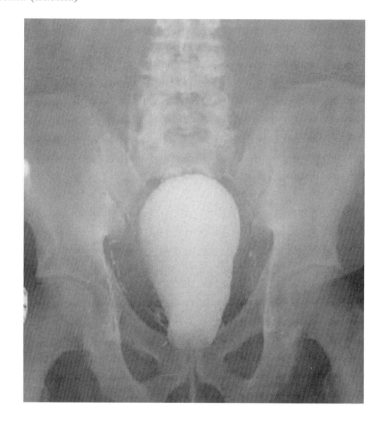

# Adrenal

## MASS

### CORTICAL

Adenoma
Carcinoma
Metastasis

### MEDULLARY

Pheochromocytoma (5 Ps)
   –pain
   –pallor
   –palpitations
   –perspiration
   –panic

## CYSTS

True—congenital
Pseudo—posthemorrhagic
Infectious—echinococcal

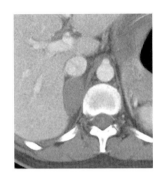

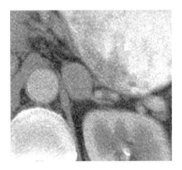

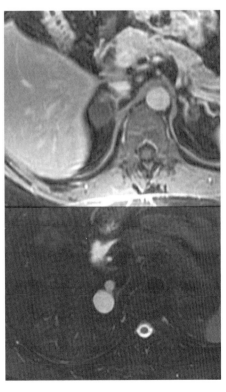

# Retroperitoneum

## NORMAL TO HEMORRHAGE

**N**eural (schwanomma, NF)
**O**rmond's disease (idiopathic RPF)
**R**PFibrosis (secondary—drug/tumor)
**M**etastasis from genital system
**A**denopathy—infectious
**L**ymphoma
**Hemorrhage**

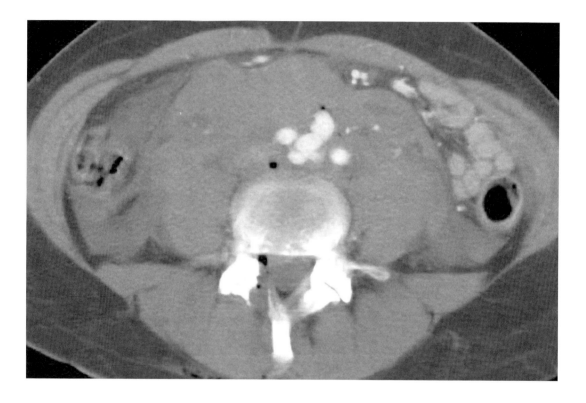

## URETHRAL STRICTURE

I[3]

    **I**nfection
        Gonorrhea
        TB
        Schistosomiasis
    **I**atrogenic
    **I**njury—posttraumatic

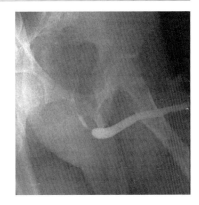

# Uterus

## HSG

Can be shown essentially two types of cases with abnormalities:
Uterus or Fallopian tube

### *Uterine Cavity*
Bicornuate vs Septate

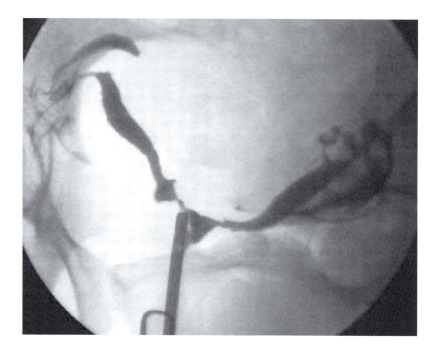

## Chapter 4 / Genitourinary Radiology

### Didelphys

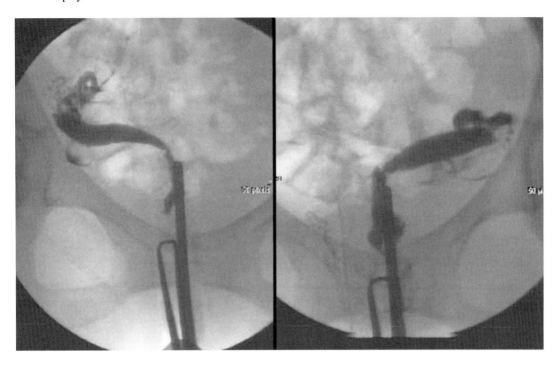

### DES

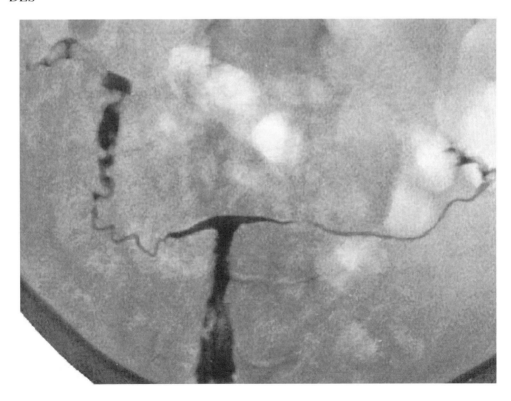

Asherman's Syndrome
Adenomyosis

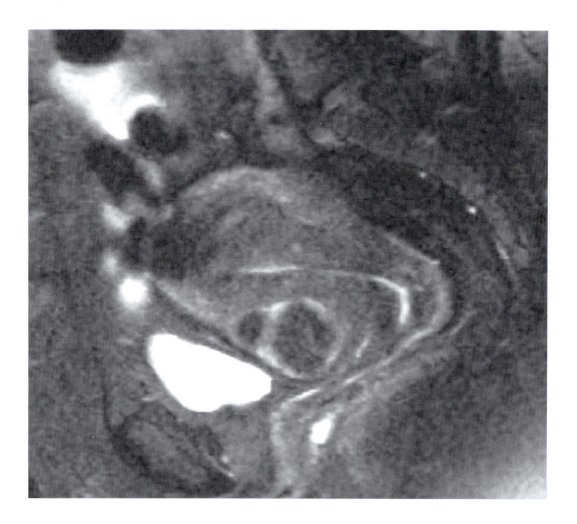

Chapter 4 / Genitourinary Radiology

## *Fallopian Tube*
Salpingitis Isthmica Nodosa
TB
Obstruction

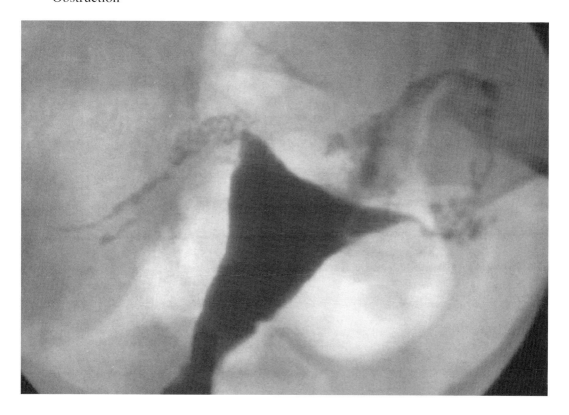

# Prostate

## CYSTS

### *Midline*

#### "U" CYST

Utricle

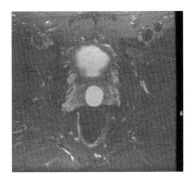

Urethra (connected)

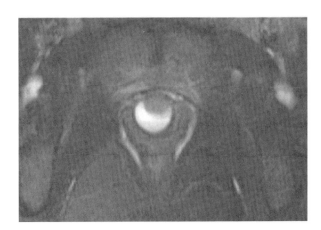

Urethral polyp association
Undescended testicle association

#### "S" CYST

**M**ullerian
**S**perm containing
**S**tone forming
**S**uperior extending (above prostate)

## *Paramedian*
BPH
Ejaculatory duct cyst

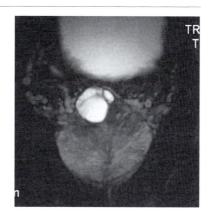

## *Lateral*
Seminal vesicle cyst (renal agenesis association)

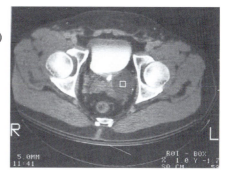

## *Infection*

## *Neoplasm*
Peripheral zone (prostate carcinoma)

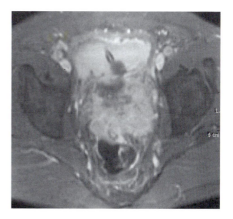

# 5
# Head and Neck Radiology

*Includes plain film diagnosis of the skull, sinuses, mastoids, spine & head & neck structures and all other imaging and special procedures related to the central nervous system head & neck. This includes angiography, myelography, interventional techniques, CT, and MRI.*

# Sinuses

## NASOPHARYNGEAL MASS
### AISLE

**A**ntrochoanal polyp
**I**nverted papilloma (destroys bone)
**L**ethal midline granuloma
**S**quamous cell carcinoma (destroys bone)
**E**sthesioneuroblastoma (destroys bone)

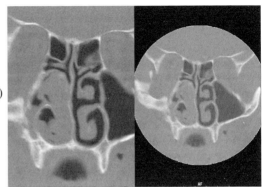

## SINUS MASS
### AFIP

**A**ntrochoanal polyp
**A**telectatic sinus
**F**ungal sinusitis
**I**nverted papilloma
**P**olyposis

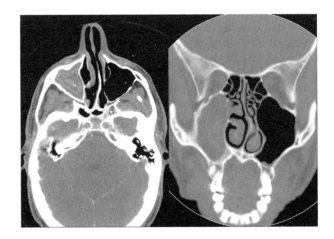

# Head & Neck Spaces

## PTERYOPALATINE FOSSA

Juvenile angiofibroma
Schwanomma
Perineural spread from V2 (palate—mouth)—adenoid-
  cystic, melanoma, lymphoma

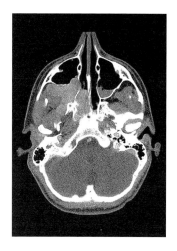

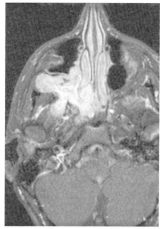

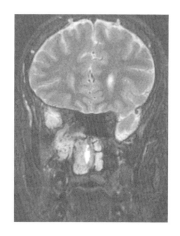

## ORAL CAVITY/OROPHARYNX

Dermoid
Ranula
Hemangioma
SCC
Minor salivary

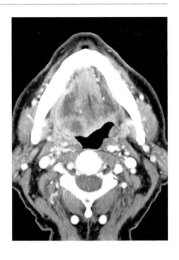

## MASTICATOR SPACE

**Bone**—Odontongenic abscess
**LN**—Lymphoma
**Muscle**—Sarcoma
**Nerve**—V3 Schwan/NF
**Mucosa**—SCC

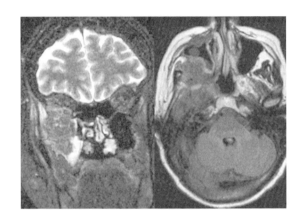

## PAROTID SPACE/PRE STYLOID PARAPHARYNGEAL SPACE

### PLEASE WATCH OUT for HEMANGIOMAS

*Benign:*

**P**leomorphic adenoma
**W**arthins
**O**ncocytoma
**H**emangioma

*Malignant:*

Minor salivary gland tumors

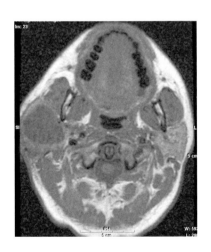

# CAROTID SPACE

**V** — Carotid body tumor
**N** — Schwannoma/NF

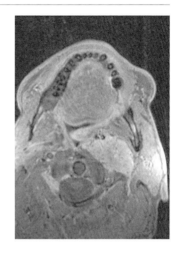

**LN** — Mets

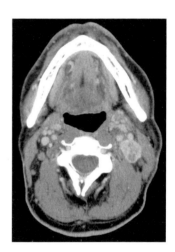

**M** — SCC

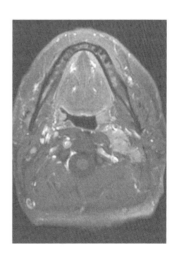

## PHARYNX

Laryngocele

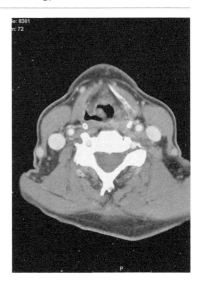

## CYSTIC NECK MASS

Second brachial cleft (fat)
Thyroglossal duct (medial)
Cystic hygroma (everywhere)
Laryngocele (pharynx)
Abscess (retropharyngeal space)
Necrotic nodes

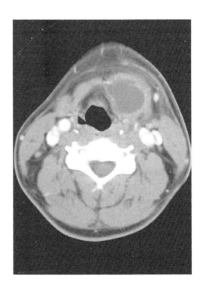

# Other

## PULSATILE TINNITUS
Glomus tumor

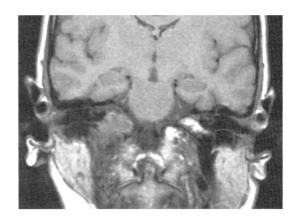

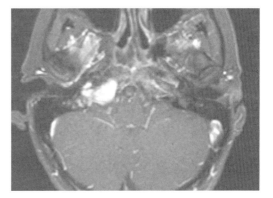

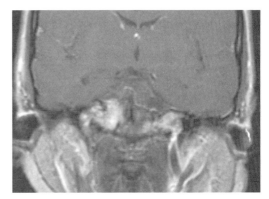

Dehiscent jugular vein (bulb)

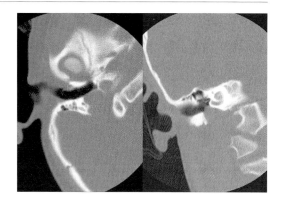

Aberrant cartoid
AVM

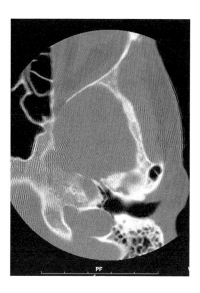

# Orbit

## LACRIMAL GLAND

### MELDS

**M**etastasis
**E**pithelial tumor—pleomorphic adenoma/carcinoma
**L**ymphoma
**D**ermoid
**S**jogrens/Sarcoid

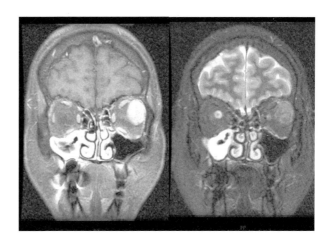

# EXTRACONAL

## LIMP + RHABDO

**L**ymphoma
**I**nfection
**M**ets
**P**seudotumor
**Rhabdo**myosarcoma

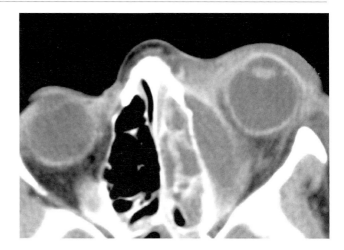

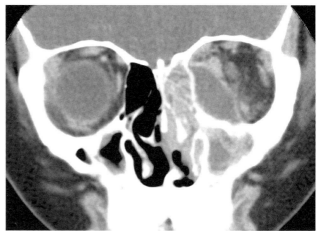

# INTRACONAL

## LIMP + HEMANGIOMA

Lymphoma
Infection
Mets
Pseudotumor
**Hemangioma**

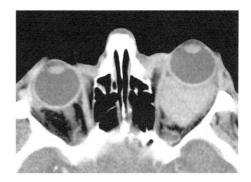

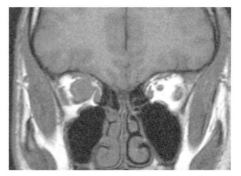

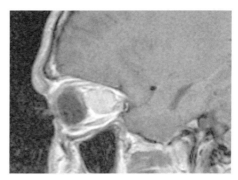

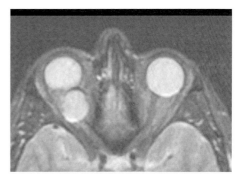

## EXTRAOCULAR MUSCLES

### LIMP + GRAVES

**L**ymphoma
**I**nfection
**M**etastasis
**P**seudotumor
**Graves**

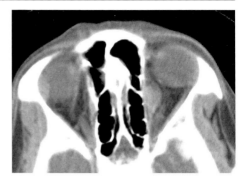

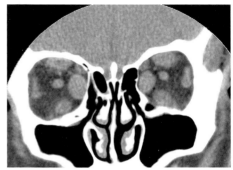

## OPTIC NERVE

### LIMP + GMN

**L**ymphoma
**I**nfection
**M**etastasis
**P**seudotumor
**G**lioma
**M**eningioma
**N**euritis

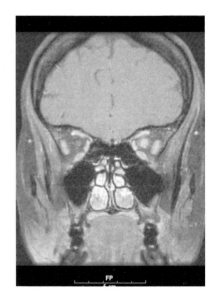

# GLOBE

Mets
Melanoma
Drusen

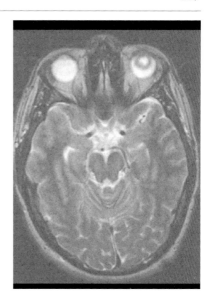

# LEUKOCORIA

Retinoblastoma
PHPV
Coats
RLF (retrolental firbroplasia)
Phthsis bulbi

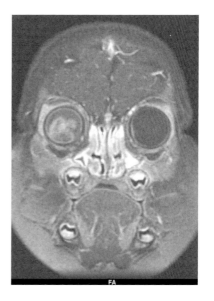

# Angle of Mandible

## ANTERIOR MASS

Submandibular gland mass
Sublingual gland mass
Larynx
Parotid

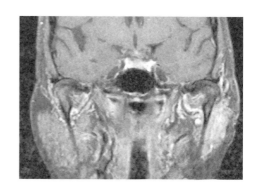

## POSTERIOR MASS (LOOK AT CAROTID)

### Splayed

Carotid body tumor

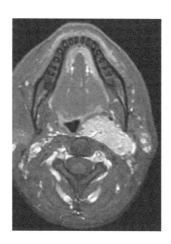
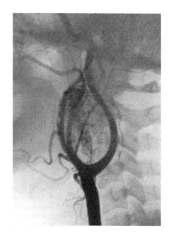

## Lateral
Brachial cleft cyst
Papillary thyroid CA
Cystic schwanomma
Cystic hygroma
Lymphoma/Node

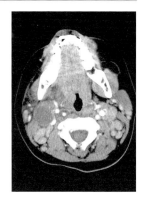

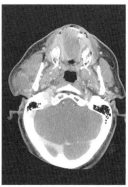

## Posterior
Node or Nerve

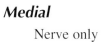

## Medial
Nerve only

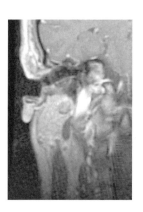

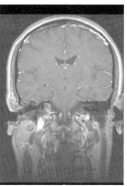

# Neck

## TUMOR
Glottic
Supraglottic (FAT)
Subglottic

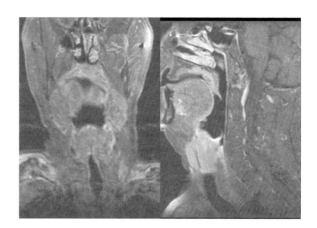

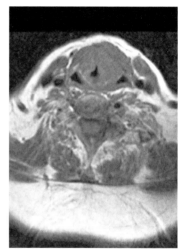

Chapter 5 / Head and Neck Radiology

# MIDLINE OR SOMEWHAT OFF MIDLINE

## *Cyst*
Thyroglossal duct cyst

## *Bone*
Chondrosarcoma

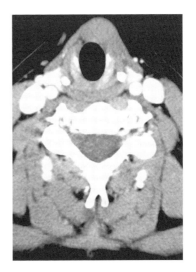

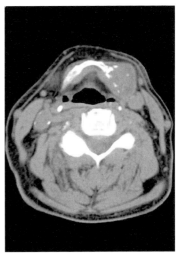

## Submucosal

Laryngocele

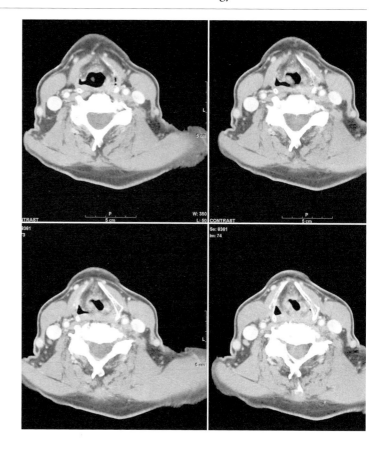

# Temporal Bone

## WHITE MASS

### Cholesteatoma
a. Tegmen tympani ? intact
b. Lat wall semicircular canal ? intact
c. Facial nerve —
   Location? Bone? Relationships?

### Cholesterol Granuloma

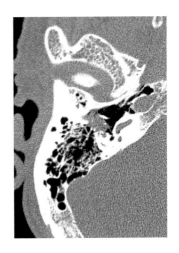

## RED MASS

### Glomus Jugulare
Erodes pars vascularis
— do angio to determine vs hemangioma

### Glomus Tympanicum
Jugular bulb ok
— no angio

### Aberrant Carotid
Peristant stapedial artery

### Jugular Bulb Anomalies

#### WORKUP
CT separates aberrant carotid/GJ/GT
MR for flow void assessment and extent

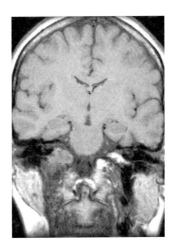

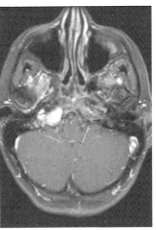

# OTHER

## MONDINI

Inner ear
Segmentation cochlear problem
Interscalar septum
Lateral semicirular canal (central post absent)
Vestibular aqueduct—bigger than posterior semicircular canal

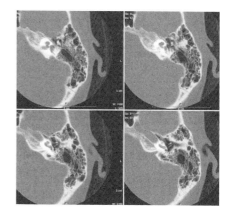

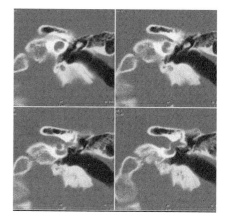

# PETROUS EXPANSION

Cholesterol cyst/granuloma T1 BRIGHT
Epidermoid/cholestetoma T1 DARK
Mucocele

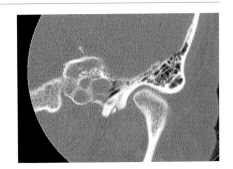
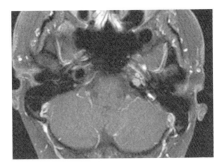
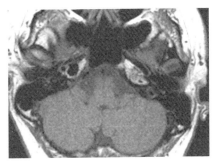

# Thyroid

## SUBACUTE

Post-viral
Hypothyorid
Fever, chills, pain

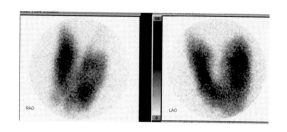

## HASHIMOTO'S

Early—Hyperthyroid

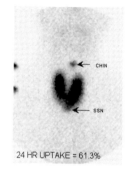

Late—Hypothyroid

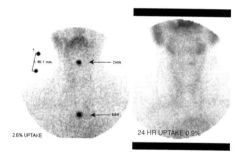

## GRAVES

Goiter
Thyrotoxicosis
Increased uptake—gland hot

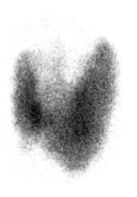

Chapter 5 / Head and Neck Radiology 157

# Skull Base

## BY LOCATION

### Midline

Craniopharyngioma
Chordoma

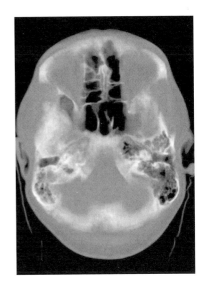

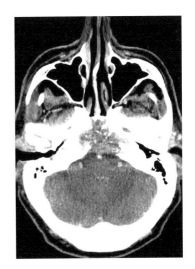

## Paramedian

Carotid aneurysm
Chondrosarcoma

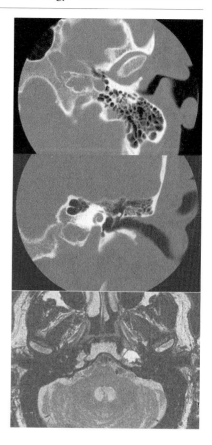

## Lateral (GW of sphenoid)

Meningioma
Metastasis
Dermoid
Glomus
Epidermoid
**Cholesterol cyst**

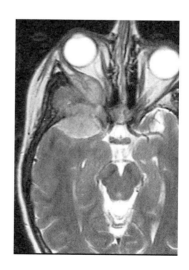

## Always Include
Mets
Myeloma
Lymphoma

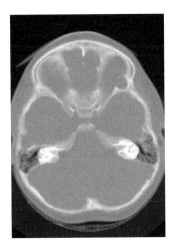

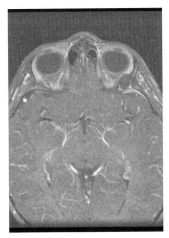
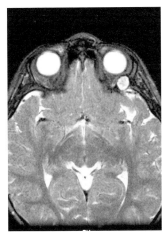

# LACRIMAL

**Epithelial**—Pleomorphic adenoma, Adenoid cystic, Mucoepidermoid
**Lymphoid**—Lymphoma, Sjogren, Benign lymphoid hyperplasia

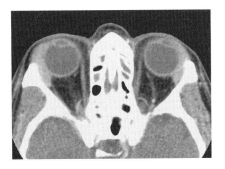

# 6
# Vascular and Interventional

*Includes the diagnosis of all abnormalities and anomalies of the arteries, veins, and lymphatics. It includes all vascular and nonvascular imaging-directed interventional procedures. All modalities and techniques used in diagnostic and interventional procedures are also included.*

## GENERAL APPROACHES

1. Technique
    a. Which vessel injected
    b. Phase of injection
        i. Arterial—early/mid/late
        ii. Venous—early/mid/late
2. Anatomy
    a. Which vessels are opacified?
    b. Are the expected vessels based on the injection filled?
    c. Are any vessels missing?
    d. Are there vessels that should not be filling?
    e. Anatomy—too small/too large/filling defects/cutoff
    f. Are there vessels that are filling early?

## TECHNIQUE SPECIFICS

### VASCULAR

*Injection and Filming Rates*

| | | | | | |
|---|---|---|---|---|---|
| Pulmonary artery | 20 cc/s | for | 40 cc | at | 8 f/s |
| Thoracic aorta | 25 cc/s | for | 50 cc | at | 8 f/s |
| Abdominal aorta | 20 cc/s | for | 40 cc | at | 6 f/s |
| Pelvic aorta/bifurcation | 10 cc/s | for | 20 cc | at | 2 f/s |
| Iliac artery | 5 cc/s | for | 10 cc | at | 2 f/s |
| Celiac artery/SMA | 5 cc/s | for | 50 cc | at | 2 f/s |
| Inferior mesenteric artery | 3 cc/s | for | 30 cc | at | 2 f/s |
| Renal artery | 4 cc/s | for | 8 cc | at | 4 f/s |
| Carotid artery | 6 cc/s | for | 10 cc | at | 4 f/s |
| Subclavian artery | 5 cc/s | for | 10 cc | at | 3 f/s |
| IVC | 20 cc/s | for | 30 cc | at | 4 f/s |

## ANGIOPLASTY

### CHOOSE

1. Diameter (usually 10% larger than the vessel)
    a. Aorta                20 mm
    b. Common iliac         8 mm
    c. External iliac       7 mm
    d. SFA                  6 mm
    e. Popliteal            5 mm
    f. Tibial               3 mm
    g. Dorsalis pedis       2 mm
    h. Renal/celiac/SMA     6 mm

# Chapter 6 / Vascular and Interventional

    2. Length
        a. Most successful for SHORT, CONCENTRIC, NON-CALCIFIED
    3. French size (for pressure measurement, sheath should be 2 FR >catheter)
    4. Shaft length of balloon
    5. Burst pressure of balloon
    6. Gradients
        a. Significant = >10 mmHg at rest, >20 mmHg after challenge
          or >10% of systolic BP

# EMBOLIZATION
## EMBOLIC AGENTS
### Liquid
- ETOH
- Glue

### Particulate
- Gelfoam slurry
- Ivalon/PVA
- Clot
- Embolization spheres

### Devices
- Coils
- Balloons

# THROMBOLYSIS
## AGENTS

| | |
|---|---|
| tPA (Alteplase) (arterial): | Infuse at 0.5–1 mg/h. Typically place 10 mg of tPA in 1000 cc of NS and infuse at 50 cc/h (0.5 mg/h). The mean time to lysis is about 20 h. The average total dose is 10–20 mg. The total dose to the patient should not exceed 40 mg. |
| tPA (venous): | Same infusion rate as arterial. |
| tPA (Alteplase) (line lysis): | Place 2 mg of tPA in 2 cc of NS and dwell in the lumen for 2 h then aspirate. |
| RPA (Retaplase): | Same as Alteplase but much more published experience with Alteplase. |
| Streptokinase: | Do not use due to anaphylactic reaction possibility. |
| Urokinase: | 100,000 U/h divided between infusion catheters. |
| This agent, however, is | no longer being manufactured. |
| Heparin: | 1000 U/h for target PTT for 60–80 s |

## Contraindications

### ABSOLUTE
Active internal bleeding
Irreversible limb ischemia
Recent stroke
Brain tumor
Left heart thrombus

### RELATIVE
History of GI bleeding
Major surgery within 10 d
Diabetic hemorrhagic retinopathy
Coagulopathy
Embolus of cardiac source

# UTLIZED MEDICATIONS

## VASODILATORS

Nitroglycerin—100 µg doses
Priscoline—25 mg doses
Papaverine—25 mg doses

## VASOCONSTRICTORS

Vasopressin—0.1–0.4 µg

## ANALGESICS/AMNESICS

Morphine—1 mg bolus, 1 mg maintenance
Versed (midazolam)—1 mg bolus, 1 mg maintenance
Fentanyl 50 µg bolus, 50 µg maintenance

## ANTAGANOSITS

Naloxone (opioid antagonist) 1 mg IV
Flumanezil (benzodiazapene antagonist) 0.2 mg IV

## COMMONLY TESTED PROCEDURES

### Vascular Intervention

#### VENA CAVA FILTER

1. Access femoral vein
2. Place pigtail catheter at iliac confluence and perform IVC gram to determine size of IVC and renal vein location
3. Exchange for wire and IVC filter sheath
4. Deploy filter
5. Re-perform IVC gram

# TIPS

1. Right internal jugular vein approach with US guidance
2. Place small catheter into hepatic veins and perform venogram after obtaining wedge pressures
3. Using direct puncture, create a connection between the right hepatic vein and right portal vein and place a wire into the portal system
4. Dilate the tract with balloon angioplasty and deploy metallic stent
5. Determine post-procedure gradients and consider coiling varices

## *Nonvascular Intervention*

### BILIARY DRAINAGE

1. Antibiotics
2. Right lateral midaxillary approach (RIGHT SYSTEM) or subxyphoid approach (LEFT SYSTEM)
3. Chiba needle or one stick system with slow injection and retraction of needle under fluoroscopy. Repeat until bile ducts visualized
4. Exchange for guidewire and plastic catheter with passage into duodenum
5. Dilate skin and place drain
6. Confirm position by fluroscopy

### CHOLECYSTOSTOMY

1. US guidance to determine pathway that is transhepatic to minimize bile leak
2. Use small spinal needle to access GB and in tandem insert 8 FR catheter
3. Aspirate for bile for culture and sensitivity
4. Left in until surgery or at least 3 wk to form tract

### PERCUATENOUS GASTROSTOMY

1. If ascites: Do paracentesis first
2. Indication dictates type of tube: feeding—GJ tube, drainage—G tube
3. Using US guidance, determine left edge of liver and spleen
4. Cup of barium from night before to outline colon through NG tube
5. Insufflate stomach
6. Gastropexy with T-tacks and retract the stomach to the abdominal wall in the high gastric body
7. Place needle between the 4 T-tacks with placement of a stiff wire into the stomach
8. Dilate skin and place peel-away sheath.
9. Place tube
10. T-tacks removed in 3–6 wk.

### ABSCESS DRAINAGE

1. Two methods: TROCAR vs SELDINGER
2. Localize abscess under CT or US guidance.
3. TROCAR:
    a. Access abscess with small spinal needle and aspirate pus for microbiology
    b. Adjacent to spinal needle, in tandem, place catheter

4. SELDINGER:
   a. Use one stick needle and place into abscess
   b. Place wire through sheath
   c. Dilate tract
   d. Place drainage catheter
   e. Aspirate abscess for microbiology

## PERCUTANEOUS NEPHROSTOMY

1. In the prone position, locate the kidney under US guidance.
2. Place a small spinal or equivalent needle in the upper pole calyx
3. Infuse a small amount of dilate contrast
4. Using a second one stick system, access the middle pole calyx under fluoroscopic guidance
5. Place wire into collecting system
6. Dilate skin
7. Place PCN tube

# GENERAL VASCULAR DIFFERENTIAL DIAGNOSIS
## AV TIMER

Atherosclerosis
Vasculitis
    a. Large vessel: GIANT/TAKAYASU
    b. Medium vessel: BERGER/BEHCET
    c. Small vessel: CTD–SCLERODERMA LUPUS
Trauma (Dissection)
Infection
Metabolic (Diabetes) or Meds (Ergots)
External (Tumor)
Radiation

## TUMOR DESCRIPTORS
### NAP IN BED
**N**eovascularity
**A**V shunting
**P**uddling
**B**lush
**E**ncasement
**D**isplacement of normal vessels

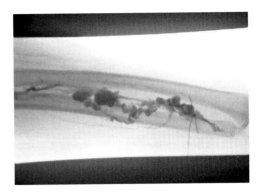

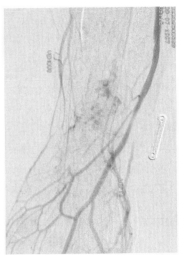

## SMALL AORTA

Williams Syndrome
Takayasu (<40), giant cell arteritis (>40)
Small aorta syndrome (female) (smoker)
Dissection
Neurofibromatosis

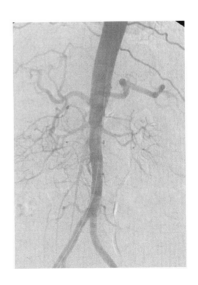

Chapter 6 / Vascular and Interventional

## POPLITEAL ENTITIES

### Intrinsic

Thrombus (popliteal aneurysm)
Embolus
Trauma

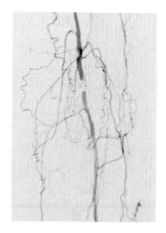

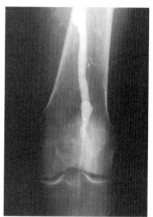

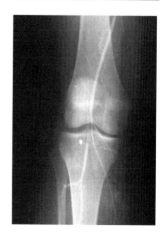

## *Extrinsic*

Popliteal entrapment syndrome

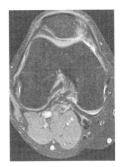

Cystic adventitial disease (MRI Dx)

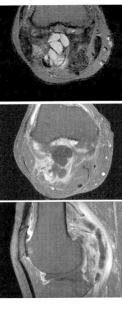

External tumor

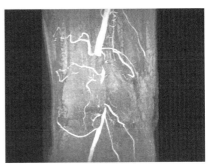

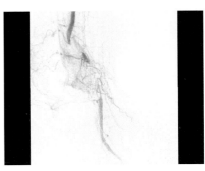

# RENAL

## Aneurysms

Polyarteritis nodosa
Lupus
Scleroderma
Wegeners
HIV
Drug-induced

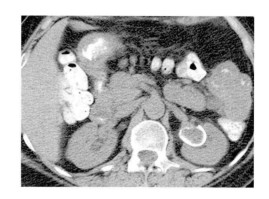

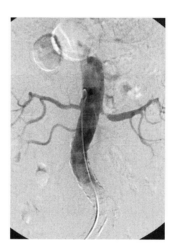
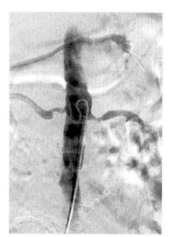

## Artery

Atherosclerosis
FMD (renal, ICA, illiac, viscerals)
NF
Arteritis
Radiation
Dissection

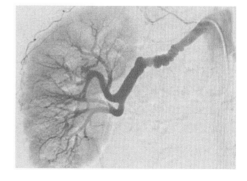

# AORTIC ROOT

## *Aneurysm*

Connective tissue disease (involves the root)
Atherosclerosis (look at the rest of the aorta)
Trauma
Vasculitis
Mycotic
Syphillis (Luetic)

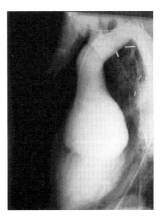

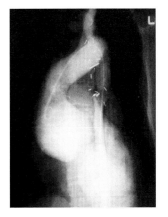

# HEMOPTYSIS

## Bronchial

Check spinal artery in field
Cystic fibrosis
Bronchiectasis
TB
Aspergillis

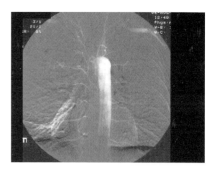

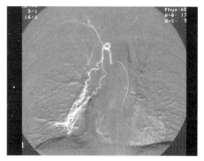

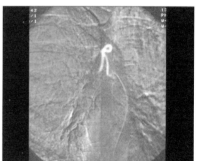

## Pulmonary Artery

Pulmonary embolus
Infarction

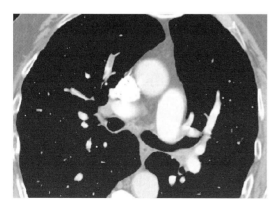
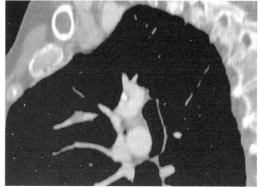

# MESENTERIC ISCHEMIA

*ARTERIAL*

*VENOUS*

Thrombotic

**Acute**  **Chronic**

*Occlusive*  *Nonocclusive*

Thrombus  Low flow  2/3 vessels occluded (Celiac, SMA, IMA)
Atherosclerosis
Surgery to resect dead bowel

GO TO SURGERY  TRY PAPAVERINE CHALLENGE

## ENDPOINTS

Ischemia to bleeding
Decompensates—peritoneal signs
Improve and wean
Heparin drip with thrombolysis

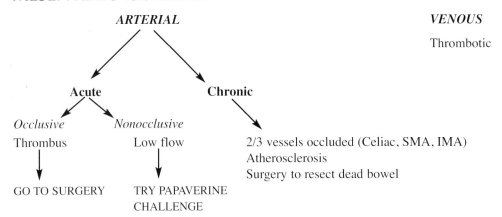
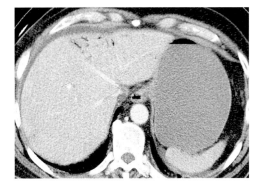
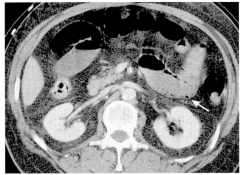
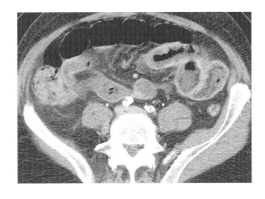

# GI BLEEDING

| UGI (Proximal To Ligament of Treitz) | | LGI | |
|---|---|---|---|
| **ARTERIAL** | **VENOUS** | **SB** | **LB** |
| Gastritis | Varices | Leiomyoma | Diverticulosis |
| Peptic Ulcer | Mallory Tear | AVM | Angiodysplasia |
| Pseudoaneurysm | | Ulcer | Cancer |
| | | | Polyps |
| ↓ | ↓ | ↓ | ↓ |
| VASOPRESSIN | TIPS/SCLEROSIS | VASOPRESSIN | EMBO VS SURGERY |
| 0.2 u × 20 min | | Except AVM (surgery) | |
| Maximum 0.8 u/min | | | |
| Recheck at 24 h | | | |
| | | | |
| EMBOLIZE | | | |
| Gelfoam | | | |
| Coils | | | |

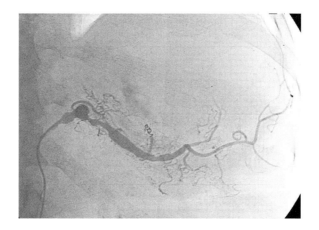

## UPPER EXTREMITY

Atherosclerosis
Thoracic outlet syndrome
Vasculitis—Raynaud's or Buerger's
AVM
Trauma

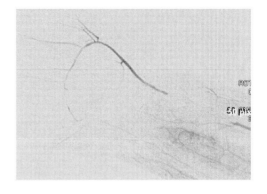

## LOWER EXTREMITY

| Viable | | Threatened | Irreversible |
|---|---|---|---|
| **ANGIOGRAPHY** | | **SURGERY** | **AMPUTATION** |
| *Embolus* | *Thrombus* | | |
| Menisci | Occlusive | Bypass | |
| Multiple | Collaterals | | |
| ↓ | ↓ | | |
| Heparin | Thrombolysis | | |
| Coumadin | | | |

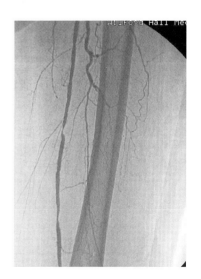

# 7
# Nuclear Medicine

*Includes radiopharmaceuticals, dynamic and static nuclear imaging of pathophysiological processes, and quality control of nuclear imaging instruments.*

# Lung Imaging

## V/Q SCAN

### Clinical
HIGH probability: 80% chance PE
LOW probability: 80% chance of no PE

### VENTILATION
1. 20 mCi Xe-133
   80 keV
   Gas
   T1/2 = 5 d
2. 4-5mCi Tc-99m-DTPA
   140 keV
   Aerosol
   T1/2 = 6 h

| | | |
|---|---|---|
| Initial phase | 30 s | –Ventilation |
| Equilibrium phase | 3 min | –Lung volumes |
| Washout phase | 3 min | –Exclude obstructive disease |

### PERFUSION
4 mCi Tc-99m-MAA (10-40 μ)
1 million particles
T1/2 = 6 h

## Defect Size
Small <25%
Moderate 25–75%
Large >75%

## High Probability
2 large/mismatched defects or the arithmetic equivalent in moderate or large defects

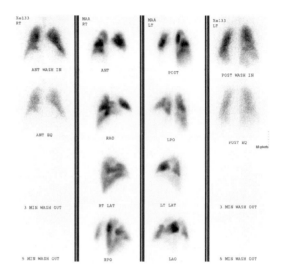

## Intermediate Probability
1 large/2 moderate mismatched perfusion defects or the arithmetic equivalent in large and moderate defects

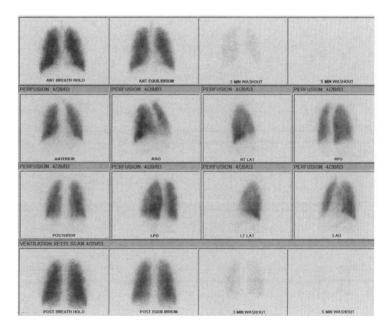

## Low Probability

>3 small defects

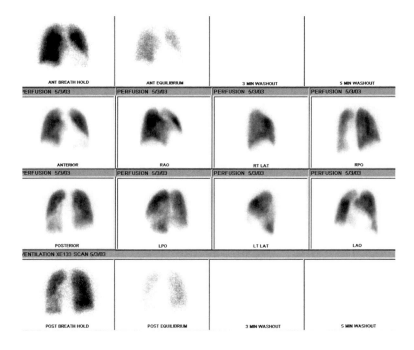

## Very Low Probability

Nonsegmental defects (i.e., cardiomegaly, prominent hila, enlarged aorta), >2 matched defects

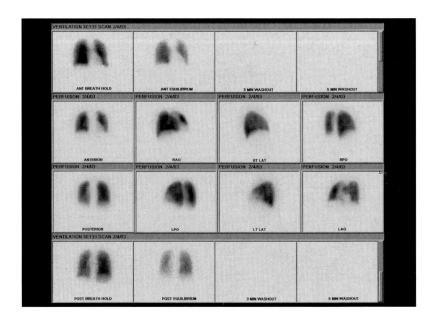

# V/Q MISMATCH
## DDX
1. Primary vascular disease (vasculitis)
2. Radiation therapy
3. PE/previous embolus
4. Lymph nodes/Hilar carcinoma/sarcoma/lymphoma

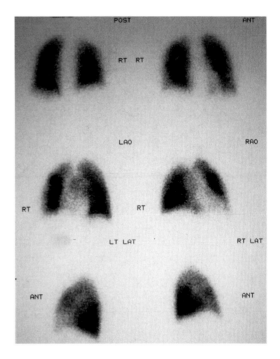

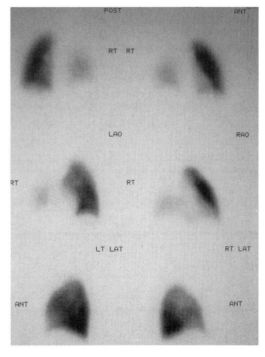

## LIVER UPTAKE

Early: Fatty liver
Late: Right heart failure

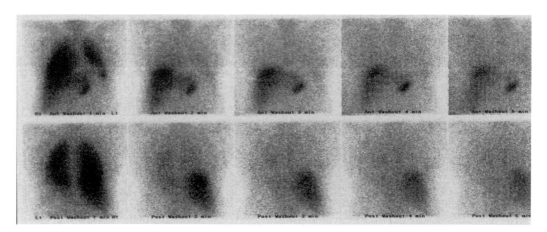

# Endocrine

## THYROID

### Approach
1. Palpable or nonpalpable nodule → nodule evaluation study
2. Clinical: Hyperthyroid? → radioactive iodine uptake study
3. Malignancy: Metastatic disease? → metastatic search

### 1. RADIOACTIVE IODINE UPTAKE STUDY
I-123
200-300 uCi
24-h uptake
N10-30%

### 2. THYROID SCAN

#### FUNCTIONAL

##### Hyperthyroid
1. Graves/Hashimoto's thyrotoxicosis
   Diffuse increased uptake

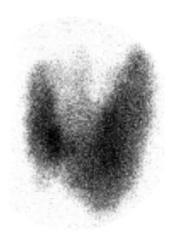

2. Subacute thyroiditis
   Diffuse decreased uptake

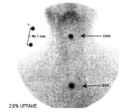

3. Toxic/Multinodular (Plummer) Nodule uptake
4. Painless, Postpartum

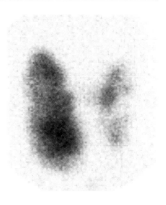

## *Hypothyroid*

Hashimoto's
Surgery
Radiation

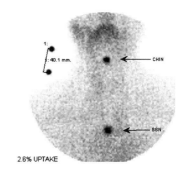

## *Nodule Evaluation*

| *I-123* | *Tc-99m* |
|---|---|
| 159 keV | 140 keV |
| 100–200 µCi orally | 5–10 mCi |
| Pinhole collimator | Pinhole or straight bore |
| Co-57 String or spot marker | |
| T1/2 = 9 mo | |

# SCAN PATTERNS

## 1. Normal-Diffuse Symmetric

## 2. Nodule

COLD

**CATCH PALM**

Cancer
Adenoma
Thyroidits
Colloid Cyst
Hematoma
Parathyroid
Abscess
Lymph node/lymphoma
Metastasis

HOT

Functioning adenoma
Malignancy <1% (rule out discordant)
Multiple
 -less likely malignant

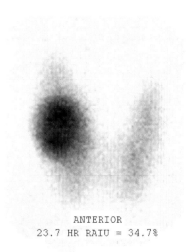

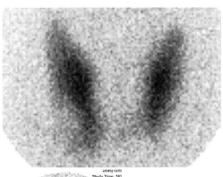

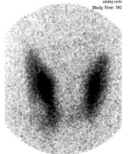

## METASTATIC DISEASE

I-131
Oral
364 keV
5–10 mCi-diagnosis
10 mCi-Grave's disease
100 mCi-Thyroid bed ablation
>200 mCi-Pulmonary fibrosis results

Normal uptake heart, stomach, bladder, stomach

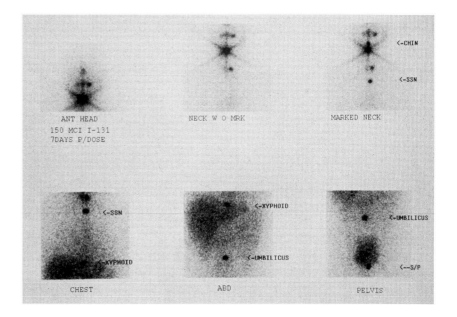

# PARATHYROID SCAN

25 mCI Tc-99m Sestamibi
DUAL WITH Tc-99m (uptake in heart is a clue)
Uptake only in abnormal glands (>35–50 g)

Parathyroid adenoma-single site

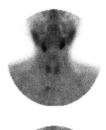

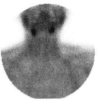

Parathyroid hyperplasia-multiple sites

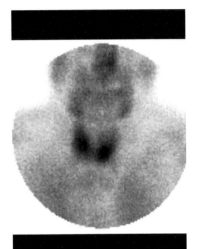

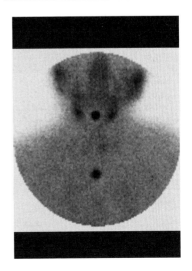

# Cardiac Imaging

## 1. VIABILITY
- THALLIUM
- PET

## 2. ISCHEMIA
- GATED
- PLANAR

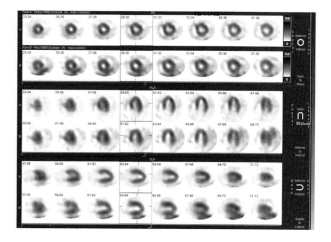

Normal

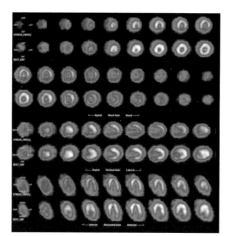 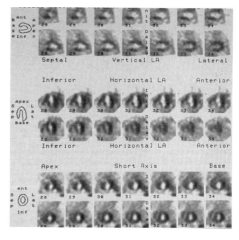

Ischemia

# 3. VENTRICULAR FUNCTION

- FIRST PASS
- MUGA

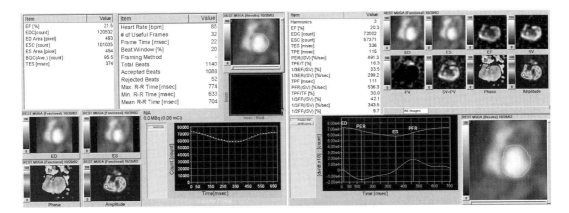

## CARDIAC PERFUSION

## PROTOCOLS

1. Thallium-201
    Rest
        4 mCi
        T1/2 = 3 d
        70 keV (Hg X-rays)
        15 min post-injection imaging
    Exercise
        20 mCi    Tc-99m-MIBI
        45 min post-injection/exercise imaging to allow clearance of liver
2. Alternates
    2 Step MIBI 8 Mci/24 Mci doses
    Tc-99m Teboroxime

## PHYSIOLOGY

### LAD Territory
Ant 2/3
Apex
Septum

### RCA Territory
Inferior wall
Inferior apex
Inferior 1/3 septum

### L. Circumflex
Inferolateral wall
Inferior wall (marginals)

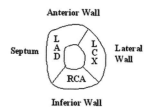

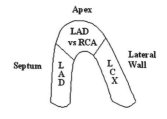

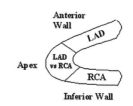

# Inflammatory Imaging

## IN-111 WBC SCAN

500 uCi
172, 247 keV
Medium Energy Collimator
Image at 24 h or 6 h/24 h
T1/2 = 3 d

### Indications
1. Fever of unknown origin
2. Infection
3. IBD F/U

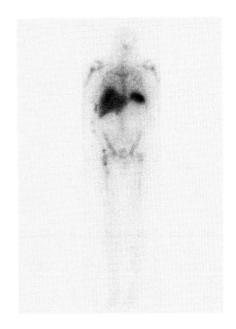

## GA-67 SCAN

5 mCi
90, 190, 290, 390 keV
Medium Energy Collimator
Image 24 h, 48 h
$T1/2 = 3$ d

### Indications

**LISA**

**L**ymphoma
**I**nfection (Lung)(MAI)
**S**arcoid
**A**bscess

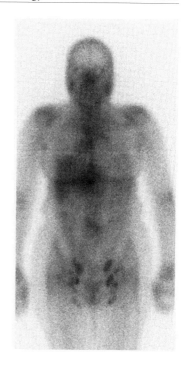

### INFECTION/INFLAMMATORY DDX

1. Lung-sarcoid
2. Lung-Pneumonitis
3. Abscess/Cellulitis/Osteomyelitis

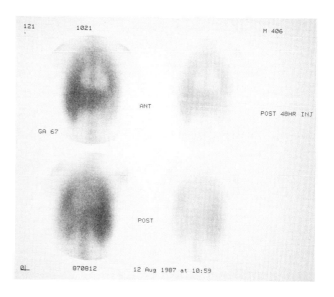

## TUMOR DDX

1. Lymphoma
2. HCC
3. Sarcoma
4. Melanoma
5. Testicular Carcinoma

    NB: No Uptake in KAPOSI

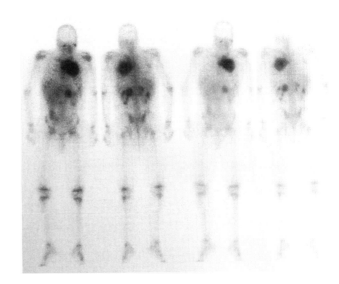

# Neurological Imaging

## BRAIN SCANNING

Tc99m HMPAO
Tc-99m ECD
20 mCi
140 keV
T1/2 = 6 h

### Indications
1. Stroke–defect
2. Dementia
3. Epilepsy
4. Brain death
5. Tumor
   Tl-201 (will see Orbit uptake)
   a) Lymphoma (+) vs Toxo (–)
   b) Tumor (uptake) vs Necrosis (no uptake)

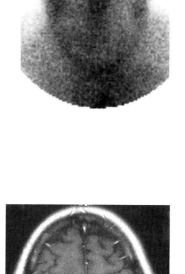

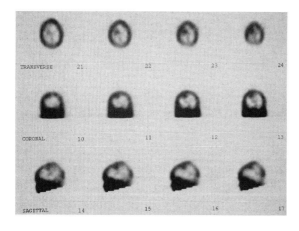

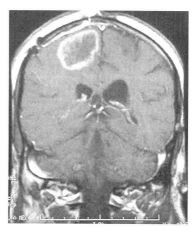

# CSF

In-111 DTPA
500 uCi
174/247 keV

## Indications

1. Dementia–NPH-immed/4 h/24/48 h
   - Early filling with reflux into ventricles abnormal (no normal reflux into ventricles)
   - Delayed clearance

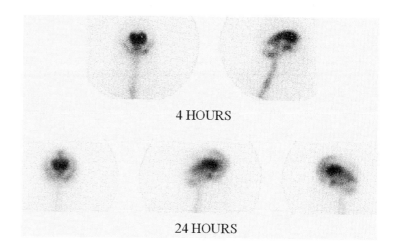

2. CSF LEAK

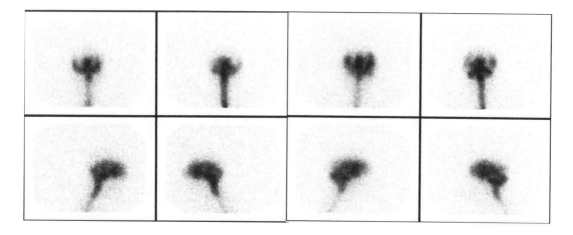

3. CSF SHUNT

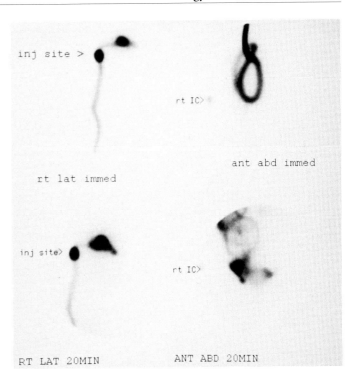

# Gastrointestinal Imaging

## GALLBLADDER/LIVER

Tc-99M DISIDA
Tc-99m MEBROFENIN
5 mCi
NPO after midnight
Q5 min × 60 min, then Q1min/frame
All purpose collimator
T1/2 = 6 h

### Evaluation

1. Does the patient have a gallbladder?
2. Prompt hepatic uptake? Peak uptake? Distribution?
3. Appropriate blood pool washout?
4. Prompt excretion into intra and extra hepatic ducts?

## POTENTIAL SCENARIOS

### 1. Bile Duct Obstruction

Normal state:

| | |
|---|---|
| Uptake in liver | 5-10 min |
| CBD | 10 min |
| GB | 60 min |
| Intestinal | 60 min |

Any delay beyond this is indicative of obstruction

### 2. Acute Cholecystitis

Augment study by giving:

Morphine 0.04 mg/kg
Sincalide 1–2 μg slow i.v. 30 min
Delay 4–6 h

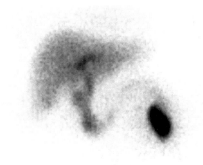

### 3. Biliary Atresia

**ANTERIOR
4 HR**

**ANTERIOR
24 HR**

## 4. Biliary Leak

Cystic duct remnant
Choledochocele
Bowel

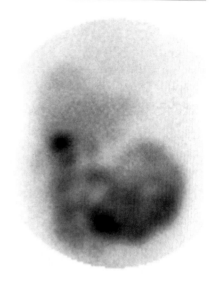

## 5. GB Ejection Fraction

Sincalide 0.02 µg/kg
    a. Dyskenesia
    b. Normal = >30% at 30 min

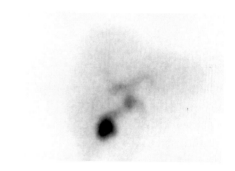

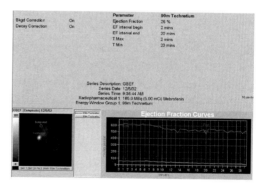

## LIVER/SPLEEN

Tc-99m Sulfur colloid
4 mCi
20 min after injection
All purpose
Planar images

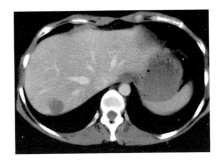

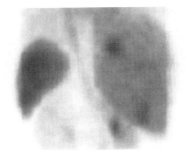

## GI BLEEDING

Tc-99m Sulfur colloid 8 mCi
Tc-99m Pertechnate labeled RBC 20 mCi
Q1 min/1 h
Requires active bleeding

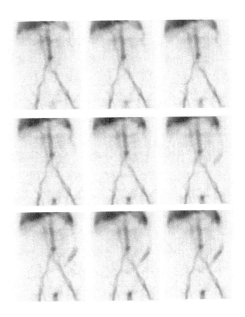

# GASTRIC EMPTYING

Tc-99m Sulfur colloid 0.5 mCi

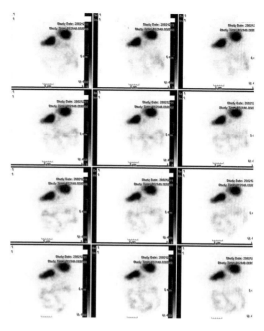

| | | Parameter | 99m Technetium |
|---|---|---|---|
| Bkgd Correction | On | Emptying | 14 % |
| Decay Correction | On | Emptying begin (T0) | 0 mins |
| Geometric Mean | On | Emptying end | 89 mins |
| | | T 1/2 | 421 mins |
| | | T0 -> T 1/2 | 421 mins |

Series Description: Gastric Dynamic
Series Date: 12/11/02
Series Time: 8:43:20 AM
Radiopharmaceutical 1: 37.0 MBq (1.00 mCi) Sulfur Colloid
Energy Window Group 1: 99m Technetium

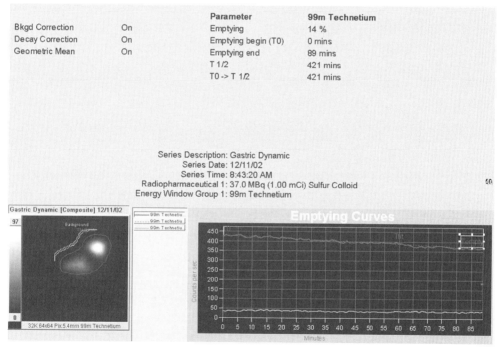

# Neuroendocrine Imaging

## I-123/I-131 MIBG SCAN

5 mCi (I 123)
0.5-1mCi (I131)
24-h imaging
159/364 keV
Low count images due to dose
Normal uptake in bladder,
    thyroid (if not blocked),
    heart, stomach, liver, spleen
No bone uptake
Abnormal uptake in other regions

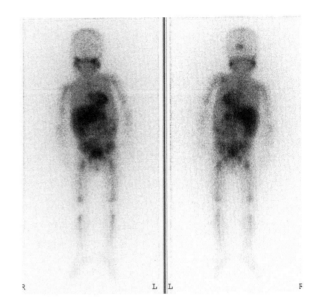

# I-111 PENTRETOTRIDE/OCTREOTRIDE SCAN

Uptake in liver, spleen, and both kidneys
Whole body images obtained
5 mCi
24-h imaging
172/247 keV
Primarily used for carcinoid and endocrine tumors

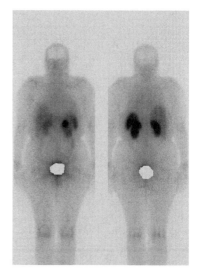

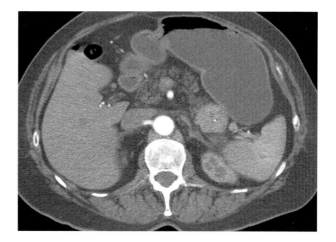

# Renal Imaging

## RENAL SCAN

Tc-99m MAG 3: 5 mCi
Tc-99m DTPA: 15 mCi
Tc-99m DMSA: 5 mCi

### Indications

| Nontransplant | Transplant |
|---|---|
| 1. Obstruction | Viability |
| 2. Function | |
| 3. Hypertension | |

### Evaluation

1. FLOW-Peak kidney uptake at 6 s equal to aortic uptake
2. FUNCTION
   a. Uptake
   b. Distribution
   c. Excretion (Prompt?)
   d. Symmetry
   e. Gradual washout
   f. Tracer in bladder

Lasix administration should cause 50% drop after 10 min

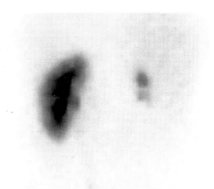

## RADIONUCLIDE VCUG SCAN

Tc-99m DTPA: 10 mCi
Reflux:
　Grade I: Ureter
　Grade II: Collecting system
　Grade III: Severe

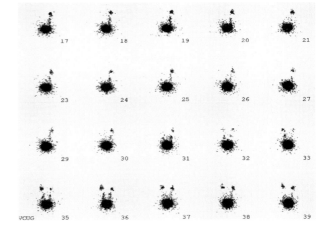

# Musculoskeletal Imaging

## SINGLE-PHASE BONE SCAN

Tc-99m-MDP: 10 mCi
3-h delay to allow soft tissue washout

### HOT FOCI-INCREASE UPTAKE

- Metastatic disease
- Tumor
- Trauma
  - Insufficiency
  - Pathological
  - Trauma
- Pagets
- Arthritis
- Osteomyelitis

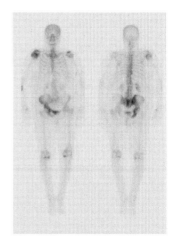

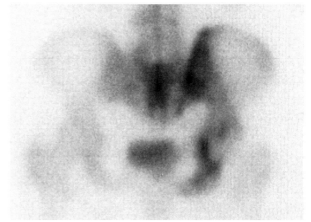

## COLD FOCI: DECREASED UPTAKE

Myeloma

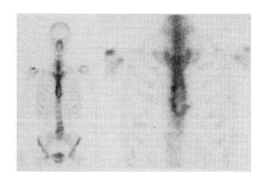

Renal cell/thyroid metastasis

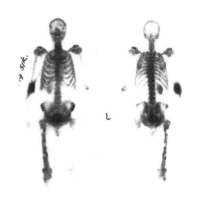

Bone cysts
Infarcts/AVN
Hardware
Abscess
Artifact

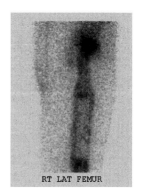

## SUPERSCAN

Metastatic disease
HPTH
Osteomalacia severe

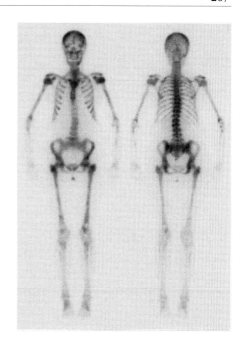

## LIVER UPTAKE

Metastatic
Previous radionuclide administration
Aluminum contamination
Amyloidosis

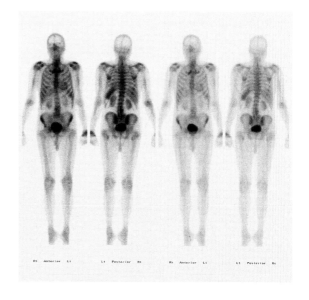

# THREE-PHASE BONE SCAN

## Indications

1. Reflex sympathetic dystrophy
   (flow at 2 mo normal, blood pool at 6 mo normal).
2. Infection

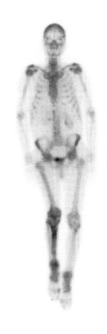

3. Neuropathic joint

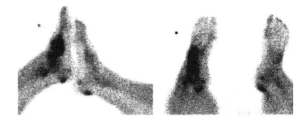

# Other

## SENTINEL NODES SCAN

100 µCi filtered Tc-99m Sulfur colloid
Intradermal injections × 4
0.1 cc/injection
Flow images at 10 s/frame × 10 min
Co-57 transmission images are combined
IMAGE ALL BEDS: Chest, Abdo, etc...
2–5 nodes typical

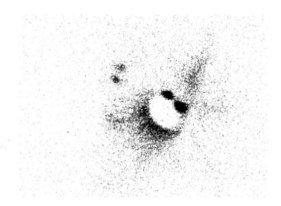

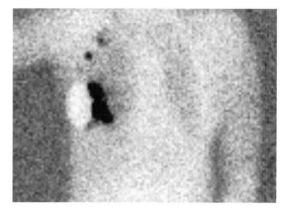

## PET

10 mCi F-18 FDG
T1/2= 110 min
511 keV annhiliation photons
Image at 1 h
Attenuation correction

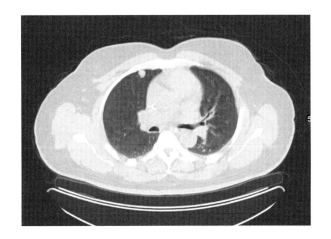

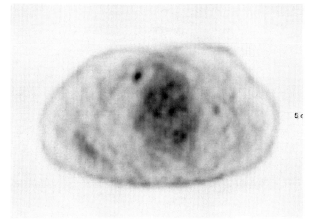

# 8
# Ultrasound

*Includes ultrasound imaging and Doppler ultrasound of the head and neck, thorax, abdomen, pelvis, extremities, breast, scrotum, and the vascular system as well as ultrasound evaluation of the fetus pregnant uterus.*

Note: Ultrasound is a different section than the other categories in that it is based on a modality rather than a subspecialty. Therefore, the cases are based on ultrasound findings rather than subspecialty entities. The following differentials are based on that principal.

# ULTRASOUND FINDINGS

## ECHOGENIC

Fat
Calcium—shadowing

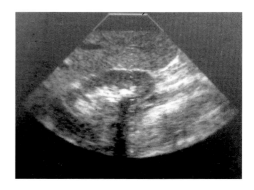

Blood

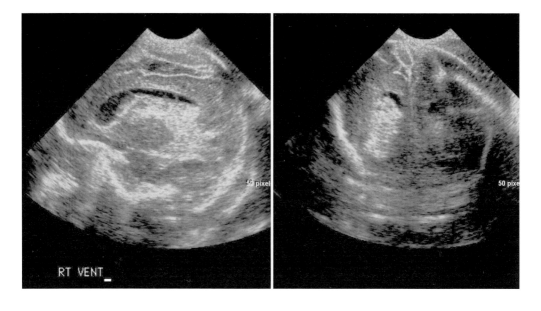

# RING DOWN OR COMET-TAIL

Cholesterol in the Rokitansky-Aschoff sinuses of gallbladder

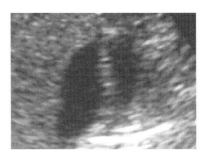

Air

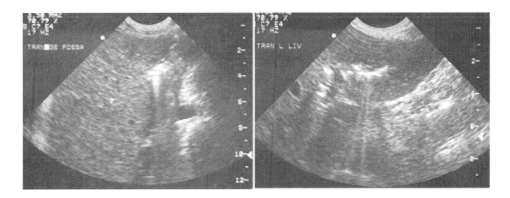

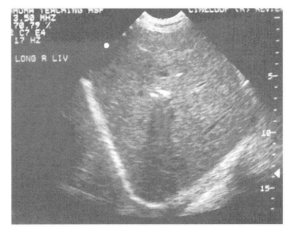

Metal

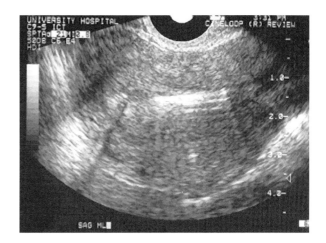

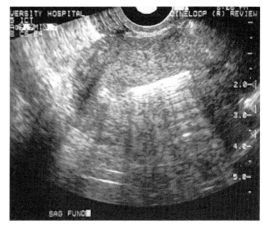

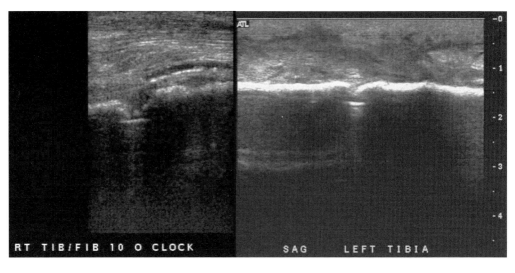

# Gastrointestinal Ultrasound

## LIVER

### SOLITARY LIVER MASS

Hepatocellular carcinoma—Cirrhosis
Adenoma—Woman on oral contraceptive
Focal nodular hyperplasia—Central scar
Cholangiocarcinoma—accompanying biliary ductal dilatation
Pyogenic abscess—Complex cystic
Focal sparing of fatty liver—Gallbladder fossa, portal bifurcation

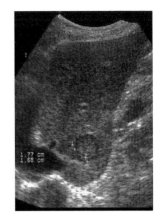

### MULTIFOCAL LIVER LESIONS

Metastases
Microabscesses—Candida
Other abscesses—Pyogenic, Amebic (complex cystic)

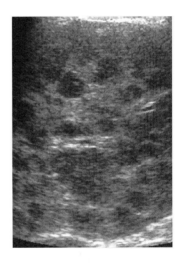

### HYPERECHOIC LIVER LESIONS

Hemangioma—MRI for confirmation
Focal fat—next to falciform ligament in anterior aspect of segment 4, portal bifurcation
Metastases—Mucinous such as colon or ovarian
Any other primary liver tumor

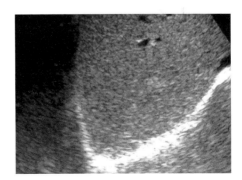

## MULTIPLE CALCIFIED HEPATIC MASSES

Stones
Histoplasmosis
PCP

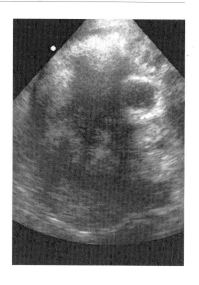

## COMPLEX CYSTIC MASS

Infection
Abscess—pyogenic or amebic
Echinococcus
Tumor
Cystic metastases—ovarian
Biliary cystadenoma
Hemmorhagic mass—e.g., adenoma (solitary)
Necrotic metastases—sarcoma
Trauma
Hematoma (solitary)
Biloma (solitary)

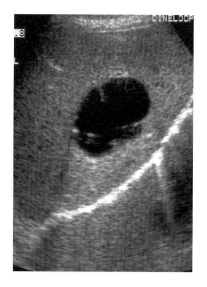

# MULTIPLE SIMPLE CYSTS

Cysts
Caroli's

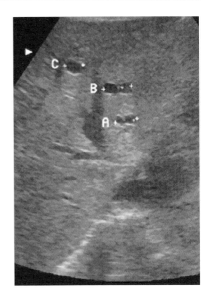

# DIFFUSE INHOMOGENEOUS LIVER ECHOTEXTURE

Cirrhosis—ascites, surface nodularity
Metastases
Fatty infiltration—loss of portal triad hyperechogenicity
Lymphoma
Kaposi in immunocompromised

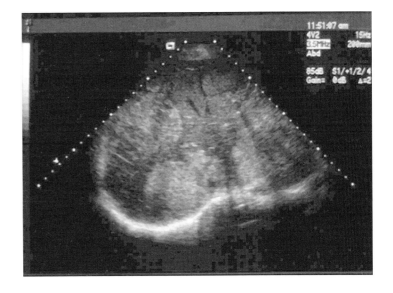

# GALLBLADDER

## SMALL INTRALUMINAL GALLBLADDER LESIONS

Stones—shadow, mobile

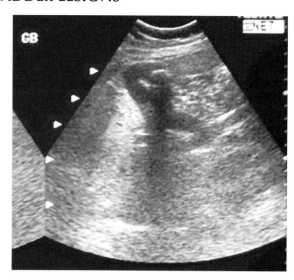

Cholesterol polyps—No shadow, not mobile

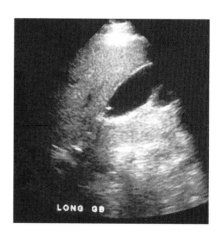

Cholesterol crystals—ring-down, not dependent

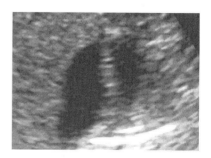

## GALLBLADDER MASSES

Polyp—<1 cm
Tumefactive sludge—mobile
Focal adenomyomatosis
Chronic cholecystitis
Gallbladder carcinoma
Metastases—melanoma

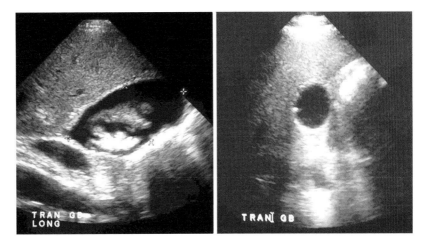

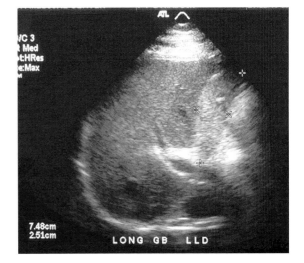

## GALLBLADDER WALL THICKENING (MANY CAUSES)

Biliary—cholecystitis, adenomyomatosis, AIDS cholangitis
Edema—hypoproteinemia (cirrhosis, nephrotic syndrome), congestive heart failure
Hepatitis

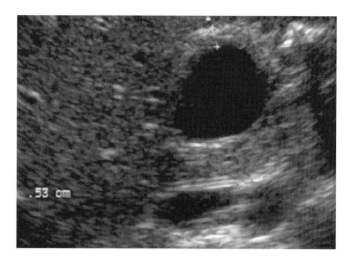

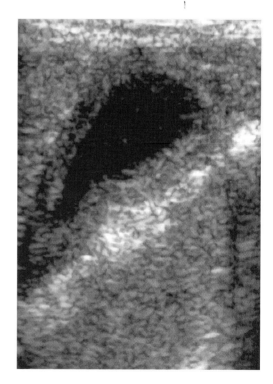

# SHADOWING IN THE GALLBLADDER FOSSA

WES of stones
Porcelain gallbladder—must be removed because of increase risk of carcinoma
Emphysematous cholecystitis

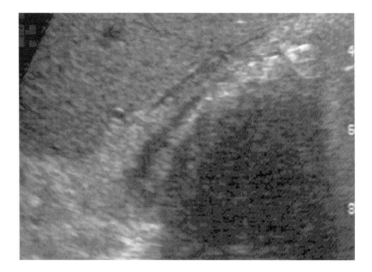

# BILIARY DUCTS

## CYSTIC STRUCTURE IN REGION OF CBD

Choledochal cyst
Duodenal duplication
Mesenteric cyst
Pancreatic pseudocyst

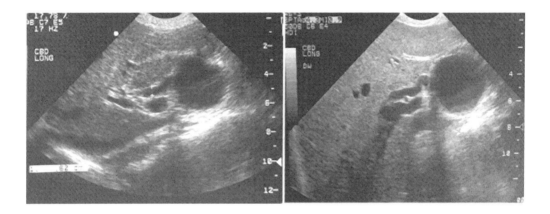

# BILIARY DUCTAL WALL THICKENING

Cholangitis
    Sclerosing—also see strictures
    AIDS cholangiopathy—looks exactly like sclerosing cholangitis
    Oriental cholangiohepatitis—stones
    Ascending
Cholangiocarcinoma
Pancreatitis

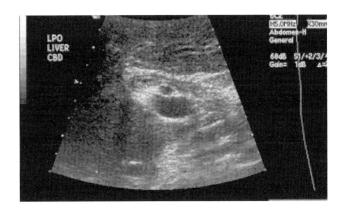

# INTRAHEPATIC BILIARY DUCTAL DILATATION

Stone
Benign stricture—chronic pancreatitis
Pancreatic head mass
Klatskin tumor

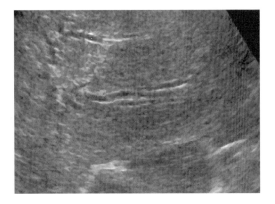

# PANCREAS

## SOLID PANCREATIC MASS

Adenocarcinoma
Focal pancreatitis—calcifications
Lymphoma
Metastasis
Islet cell tumor
Peripancreatic lymph node

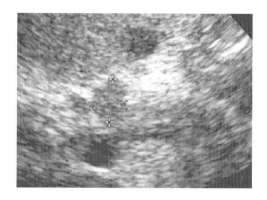

## CYSTIC PANCREATIC MASS

Pseudocyst
Macrocystic = mucinous cystadenoma/ carcinoma (middle-aged women)
Microcystic = serous cystadenoma (middle-aged women)
Solid and papillary epithelial neoplasm (young women)
IPMT—dilated side branches, 85% malignant
Aneurysm or pseudoaneurysm (pancreatitis)

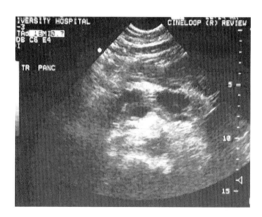

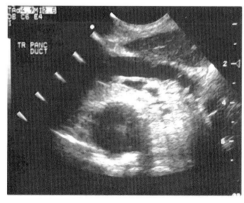

# CYST ADJACENT TO MEDIAL ASPECT OF SPLEEN

Pancreatic pseudocyst
Renal cyst

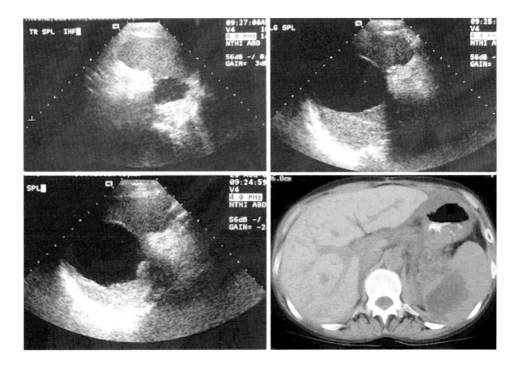

# SPLEEN

## CYSTIC SPLENIC MASS

Pseudocyst—acquired from prior trauma or infarct; most common
Epidermoid cyst—congenital
Lymphangioma
Hematoma
Abscess

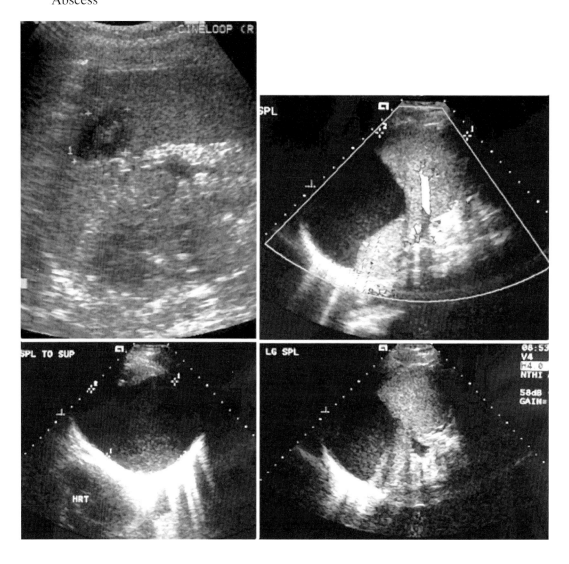

## SOLID SPLENIC MASS

Hemangioma—hyperechoic
Lymphoma—may be multiple
Infarct—wedge shaped
Abscess—Candida gives multiple microabscesses
Sarcoidosis—multiple

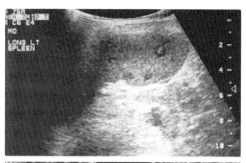

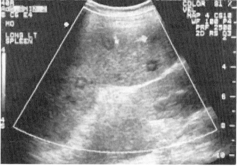

## SPLENOMEGALY

Portal hypertension
Splenic vein thrombosis
Leukemia/lymphoma
Mononucleosis
Glycogen storage disease
Myelofibrosis

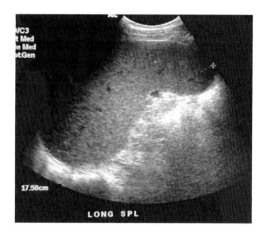

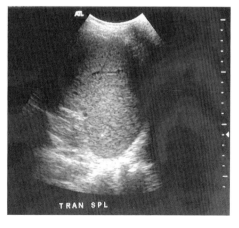

# THYROID

## THYROID MASS

### CATCH

**C**arcinoma—microcalcifications
**A**denoma
**T**hyroiditis
**C**olloid Cyst
**H**yperplasia (Parathyroid gland)

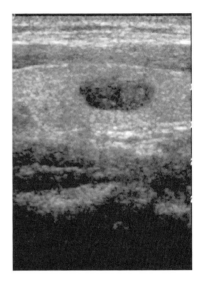

# Genitourinary Ultrasound

## KIDNEY

### HYDRONEPHROSIS

Obstruction
Reflux
Active diuresis
Congenital megacalyces

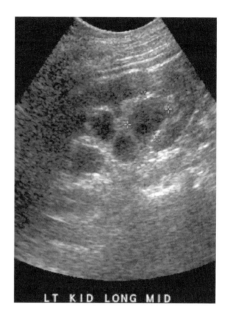

### RI >0.7

Acute tubular necrosis
Renal vein thrombosis
Obstruction
Complication in transplanted kidney = rejection, perinephric collection, cyclosporin toxicity

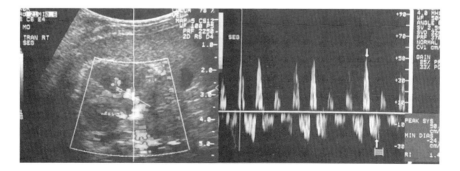

## MEDULLARY NEPHROCALCINOSIS

Renal tubular acidosis
Medullary sponge kidney
Hyperparathyroidism

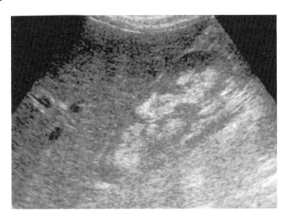

## CORTICAL NEPHROCALCINOSIS

Chronic glomerulonephritis
Healed pyelonephritis
XGP
TB

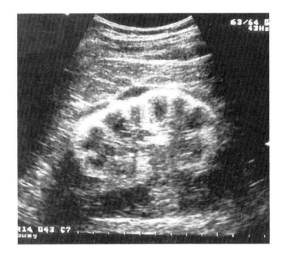

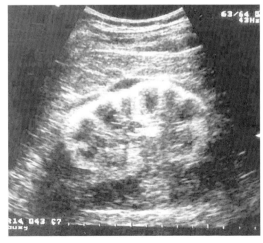

# PAPILLARY NECROSIS

## NSAID

**N**SAID
**S**ickle cell
**A**nalgesics
**I**nfection (TB)
**D**iabetes

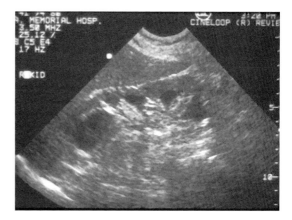

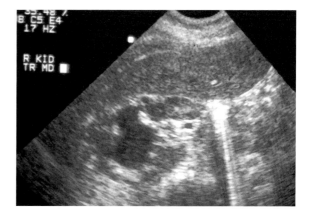

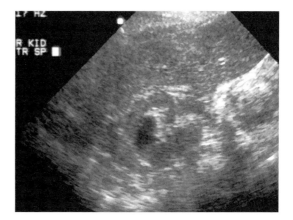

## CYSTIC STRUCTURES ADJACENT TO RENAL HILUM

Hydronephrosis
Peripelvic cysts
Papillary necrosis
Dilated renal vein

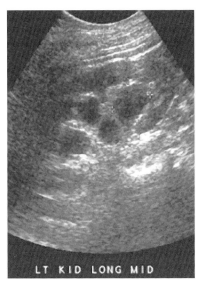

## BILATERAL MULTIPLE RENAL CYSTS

*Acquired cystic disease of dialysis* — small kidneys, increased risk of RCC
*ADPKD* — enlarged kidneys, liver cysts, berry aneurysms
*Von-Hippel Lindau* — pancreatic cysts, increased risk of RCC, CNS hemangioblastomas, pheos
*Tuberous sclerosis in kids* — AMLs, cortical tubers, giant cell astrocytomas, periventricular nodules, cardiac rhabdomyomas, pulmonary LAM

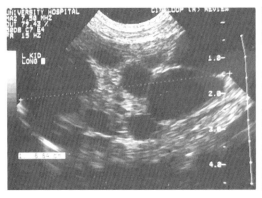
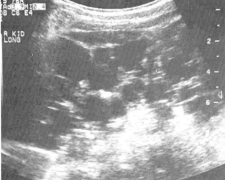

## HYPERECHOIC RENAL MASS

Stone (shadow)
AML
RCC
Lobar nephronia

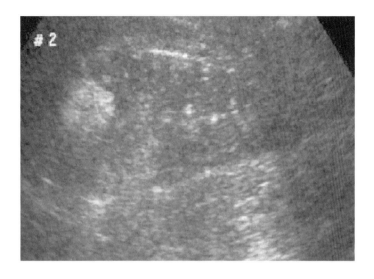

## ECHOGENIC KIDNEYS

### GLAD

**G**lomerulonephritis
**L**upus
**A**IDS
**D**iabetes

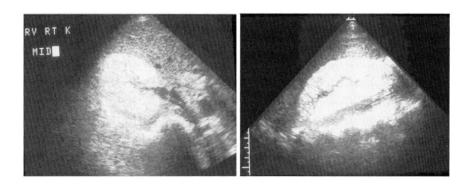

## SOLID RENAL MASS

> Tumor
>> RCC
>> Lymphoma or mets—multiple
>> AML—hyperechoic
>> Oncocytoma—central scar
>
> Lobar nephronia
> Hypertrophic column of Bertin—extend into renal sinus
> Focal parenchymal hypertrophy in atrophic kidney

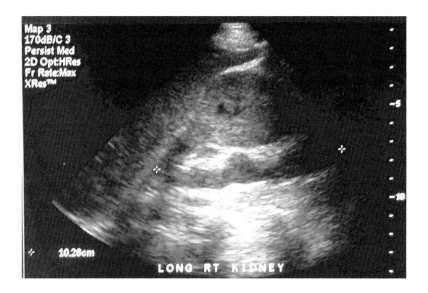

## COMPLEX CYSTIC RENAL MASS

> Tumor—RCC, multilocular cystic nephroma
> Hemorrhage into cyst
> Abscess—fever
> Hematoma—biopsy, trauma
> Hemorrhage into mass—e.g., AML

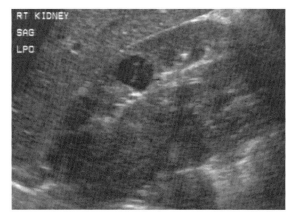

# ENLARGED KIDNEY WITH LOSS OF CORTICO-MEDULLARY ARCHITECTURE

Infection
Renal vein thrombosis
Rejection, ATN, or cyclosporin toxicity in renal Tx
Lymphoma

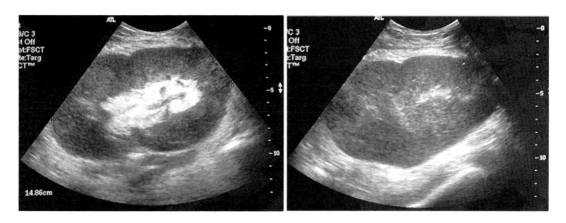

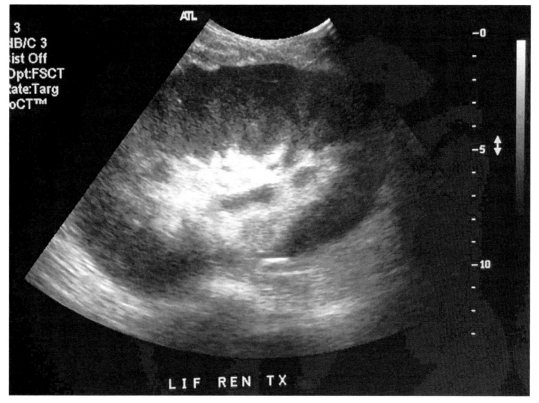

# SHADOWING FOCI ADJACENT TO RENAL HILUM

Stone
Renal artery calcification

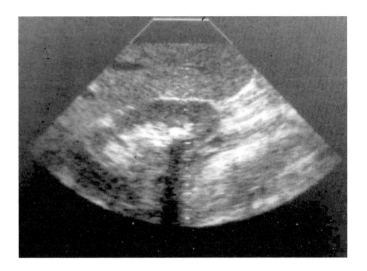

# ECHOGENIC MATERIAL IN COLLECTING SYSTEM

Stone
Clot
TCC
Pus
Fungus ball

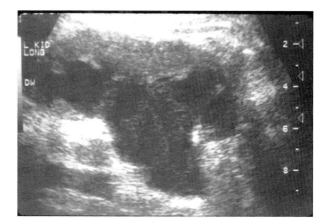

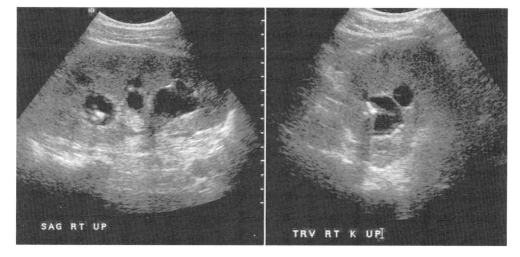

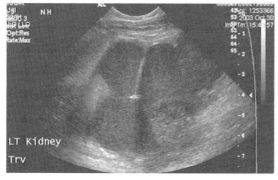

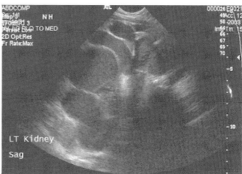

# FLUID COLLECTION AROUND TRANSPLANTED KIDNEY

Hematoma
Lymphocele
Urinoma—usually originate from ureteric implantation site into bladder
Abscess

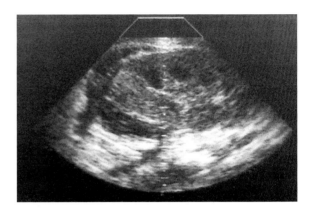

# BLADDER

## THICKENED BLADDER WALL

Bladder outlet obstruction
   Posterior urethral valves
   Prostatic hypertrophy
   Neurogenic bladder

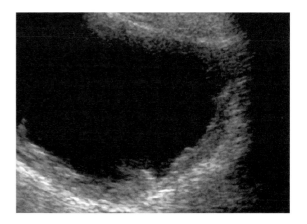

# TESTIS + PROSTATE

## INTRATESTICULAR MASS

Tumor—Palpable

    Primary malignant—seminoma, germ cell tumor
    Primary benign—Leydig and Sertoli cell
    Metastasis—lymphoma

Infection—Nonpalpable

    Focal orchitis
    Abscess

Hematoma

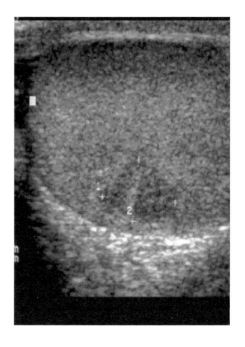

## DIFFUSELY ENLARGED HYPOECHOIC TESTIS

Torsion—decreased flow
Orchitis
Tumor—lymphoma, seminoma

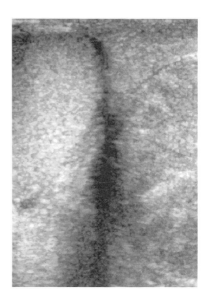

## HYPERECHOIC FOCI

Testicular microlithiasis
Microcalcifications in undescended testis
Kleinfelter's Syndrome
Sarcoid

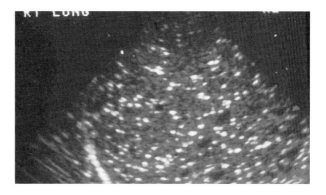

## EPIDIDYMAL MASS

Focal epididymitis
Sperm cell granuloma—post-vasectomy
Benign adenomatoid tumor

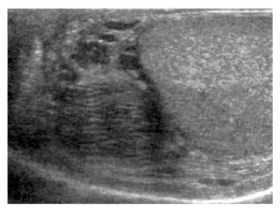

## HYPOECHOIC PROSTATIC NODULE

Malignant-Ca
Benign—prostatitis, BPH, infarct

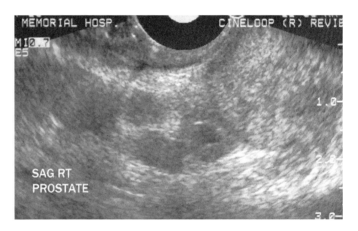

# Obstetrical Ultrasound

## UTERUS

### EXTRAUTERINE MASS WITH +βHCG = ectopic

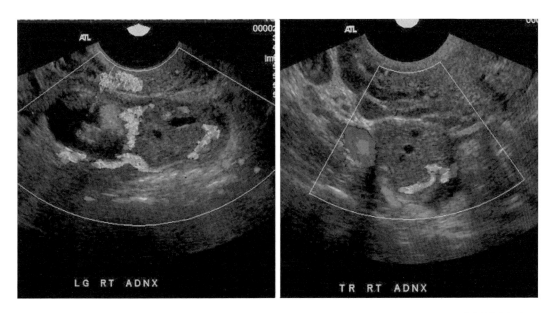

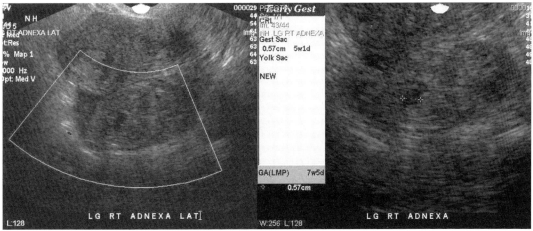

# COMPLEX INTRAUTERINE MASS WITH + βHCG

Molar pregnancy
Failed pregnancy with retained products of conception
Decidual reaction of ectopic

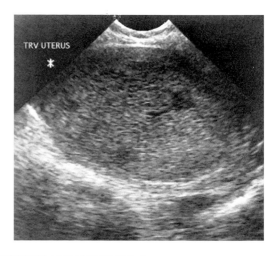

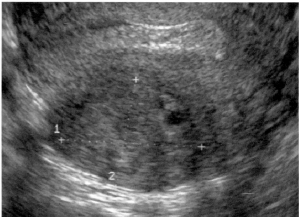

# GESTATION

## EMPTY GESTATIONAL SAC IN FIRST TRIMESTER

Normal IUP <5 wk
Ectopic with pseudogestational sac
Failed pregnancy—blighted ovum; missed abortion
1000 u/5.0 wk—GS
>1000 u/5.5 wk—GS + YS
10,000+ u/6.0 wk—GS + YS + EMBRYO

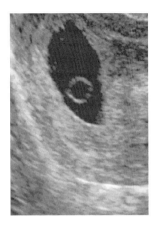

## OLIGOHYDRAMNIOS

GU anomalies—e.g., renal agenesis; obstruction
Spontaneous rupture of membranes—third trimester
Fetal demise >5 d

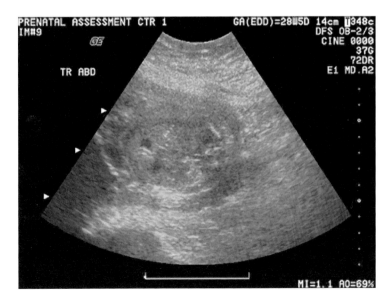

## POLYHYDRAMNIOS

Idiopathic
Maternal diabetes
CNS or GI anomalies that inhibit swallowing
Hydrops

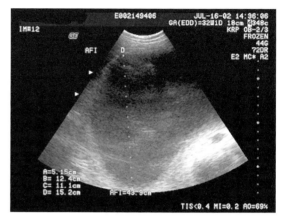

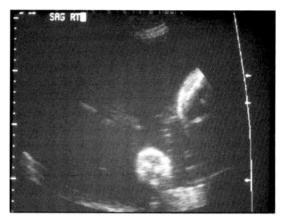

## IUGR

Placental insufficiency—hypertension, diabetes
Smoking, drug abuse
Chromosomal anomalies

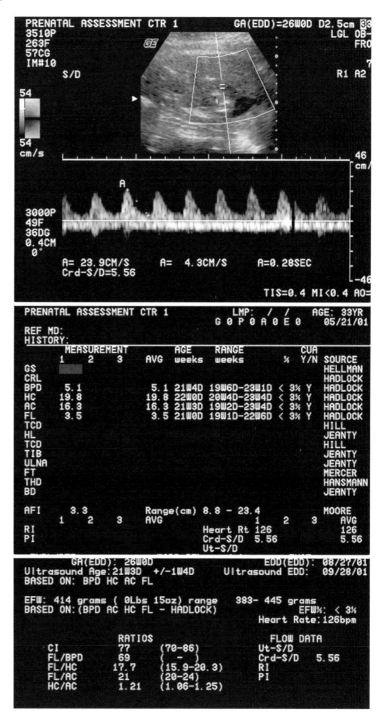

## HYDROPS

Immune (rare now with RhoGam)
Cardiovascular—arrhythmia, anatomic anomalies
Chromosomal anomalies—karyotype
TORCH infections—titers
Anemias—umbilical cord sampling
High output failure—sacrococcygeal teratoma; chorioangioma
Twin-to-twin transfusion syndrome

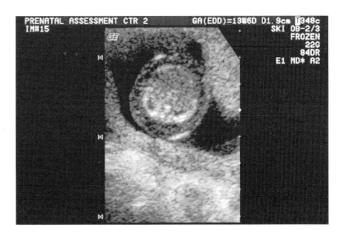

# CNS + FACE

## FLUID-FILLED SKULL

Hydrocephalus (mantle of cortex)
Hydranencephaly (irregular hyperechoic areas of tissue)

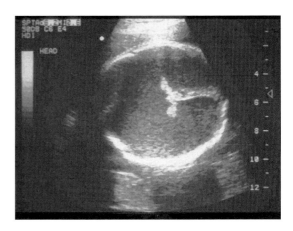

## THICKENED NUCHAL FOLD

First 11–14 wk 3 MM (IN–IN)
Second 15–20 wk 6 MM (OUT–OUT)

Trisomy 21
Turners

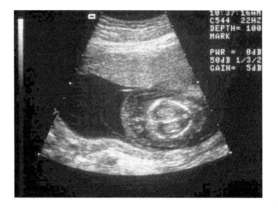

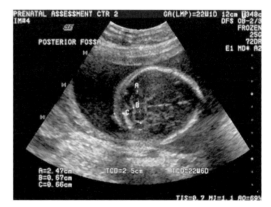

## CYSTIC STRUCTURE ADJACENT TO SKULL

Cystic hygroma
Encephalocele or myelomenigocele—calvarial defect; signs of open neural tube defect
Teratoma

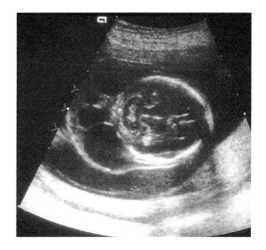

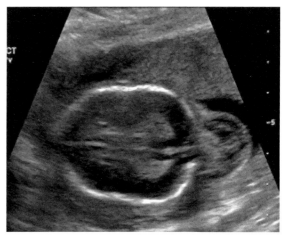

## CYSTIC HYGROMA

Chromosomes—Turner's, Trisomy 21
Lymphangiectasia
Hydrops

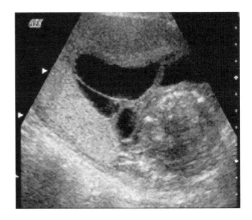

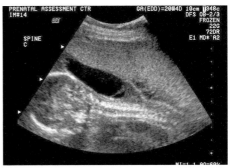

# AGENESIS OF THE CORPUS CALLOSUM/SEPTUM PELLUCIDUM

Intrahemispheric cyst
 –Colpocephaly
 –Absent cavum

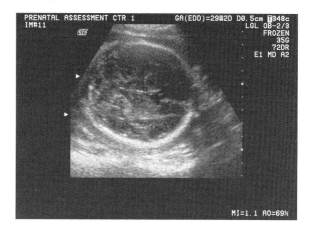

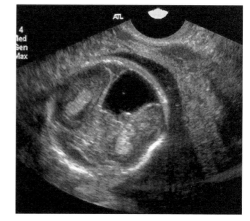

Dandy Walker
Chiari
Trisomy 13, 18

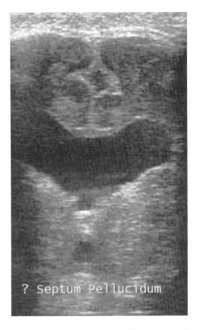

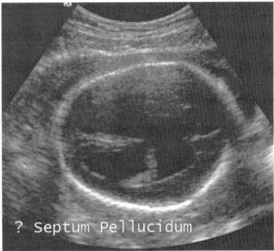

## VENTRICULOMEGALY

TORCH
Chromosomal—Trisomy 21
Intracranial bleed
Dandy-Walker, Chiari
Aqueductal stenosis

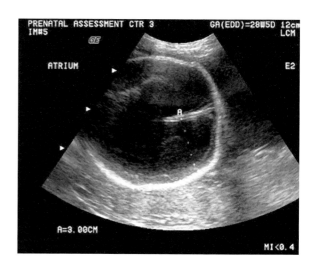

## CYSTIC STRUCTURE IN POSTERIOR FOSSA

Normal before 8 wk
Dandy-Walker malformation or variant
Mega cisterna magna
Arachnoid cyst

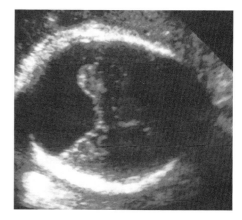

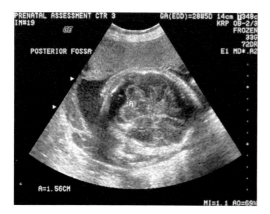

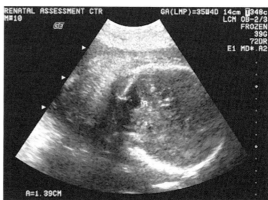

## INTRACRANIAL CYSTIC STRUCTURE

Arachnoid cyst
Porencephalic cyst

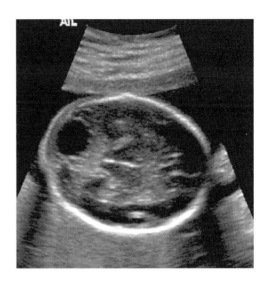

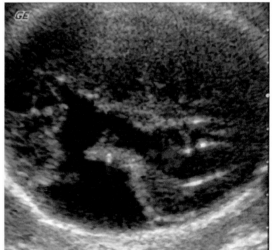

## HYPOTELORISM

Holoprosencephaly
Trisomy 13
Maternal phenylketonuria

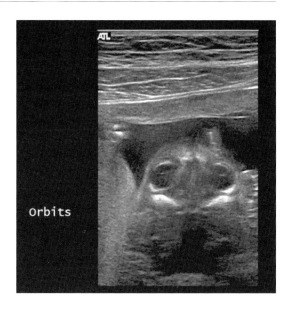

## HYPERTELORISM

Frontal encephalocele
Cleft lip sequence
Apert syndrome

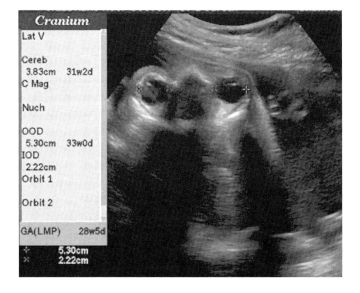

## CLEFT LIP AND PALATE

Chromosomal—trisomy 13
Teratogen—fetal alcohol
Holoprosencephaly

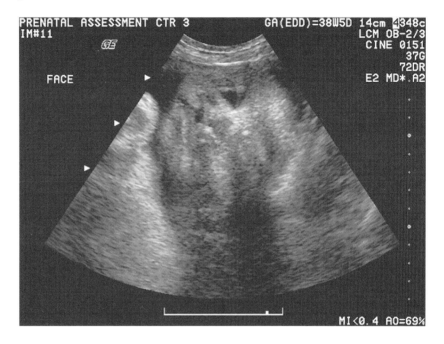

## MASS POSTERIOR TO THE SACRAL SPINE

Sacrococcygeal teratoma
Myelomeningocele (spinal dysraphism with banana and lemon signs)

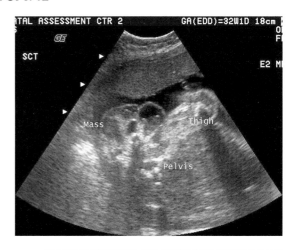

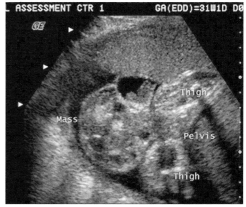

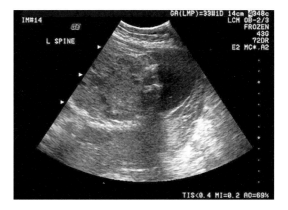

## PRESACRAL SOFT TISSUE MASS

Sacrococcygeal teratoma
Anterior myelomenigocele
Chordoma

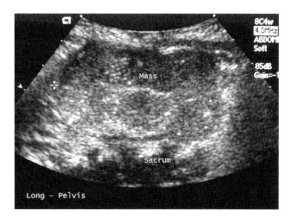

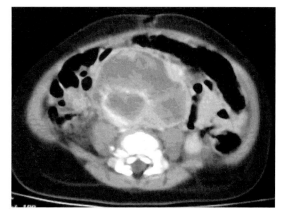

# CHEST

## CYSTIC MASS IN THE CHEST

CCAM I or II
Diaphragmatic hernia
Bronchopulmonary foregut malformation,
    e.g., bronchogenic cyst, esophageal duplication
Teratoma

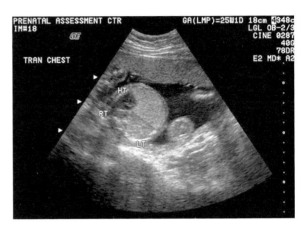

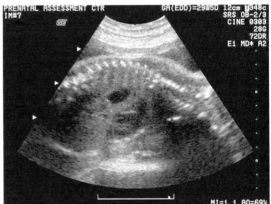

# SOLID MASS IN THE CHEST

Pulmonary sequestration
CCAM III
Morgagni diaphragmatic hernia (liver herniation)

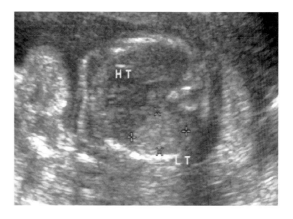

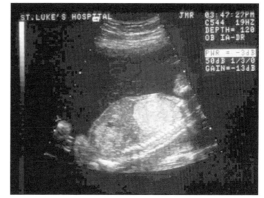

## PLEURAL EFFUSION

Hydrops—bilateral
Chylous—unilateral

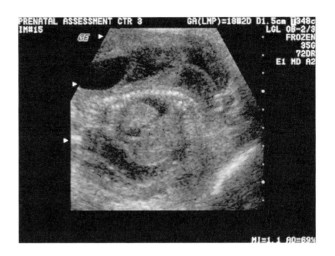

# ABDOMEN

## ANTERIOR ABDOMINAL WALL DEFECT

Normal prior to 12 wk

Omphalocele—covered by membrane; associated with structural and chromosomal anomalies

Gastroschisis—free-floating bowel; no associated anomalies

Bladder or cloacal extrophy = omphalocele, imperforate anus, myelomeningocele

Amniotic bands

Pentalogy of Cantrell—ecotopia cordis; omphalocele

Limb–body wall complex—neural tube defect, limb anomalies, short straight umbilical cord

Beckwith-Wiedemann = omphalocele, macroglossia, visceromegaly

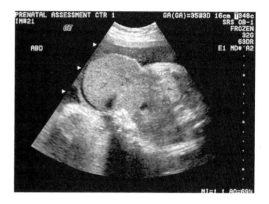

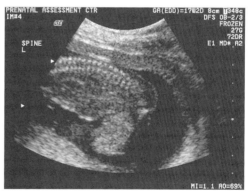

## CALCIFICATIONS IN ABDOMEN

Meconium peritonitis
TORCH
Calcified teratoma
Echogenic bowel (no shadowing)

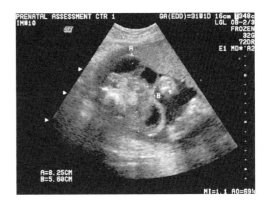
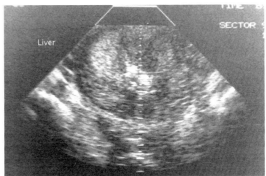
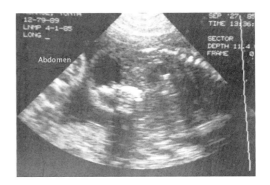
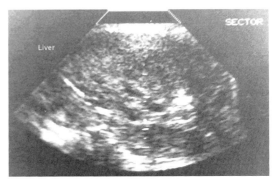

## MECONIUM PERITONITIS—CALCIFICATIONS; CALCIFIED PSEUDOCYST

Normal
Distal obstruction
—atresia, volvulus, polyhydramnios
Cystic fibrosis—meconium ileus

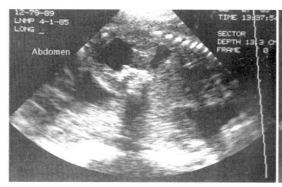
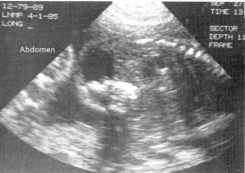
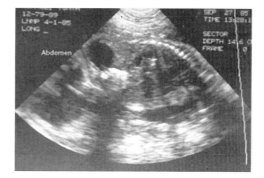

## ABSENT STOMACH BUBBLE

Esophageal .
Diaphragmatic hernia
CNS anomaly causing absence
　of swallowing
Oligohydramnios

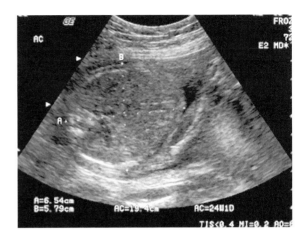

## DOUBLE BUBBLE

Duodenal atresia—Trisomy 21
Annular pancreas
Malrotation with midgut volvulus
Choledochal cyst

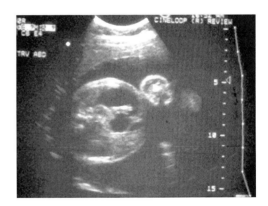

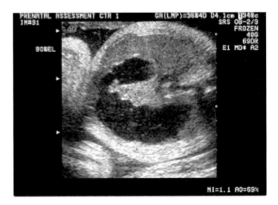

## CYSTIC STRUCTURE IN ABDOMEN AND PELVIS WITH NORMAL STOMACH BUBBLE

Renal cysts, hydronephrosis, urinoma
Bladder
Bowel duplication
Ovarian cyst
Mesenteric cyst
Urachal cyst
Teratoma

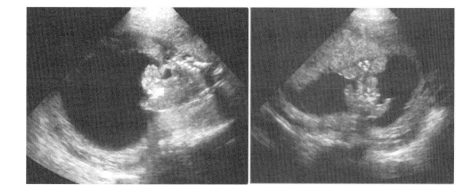

# LIVER

## CALCIFICATIONS IN LIVER

Incidental
TORCH—esp. CMV or Toxoplasmosis

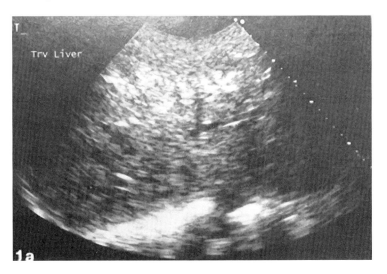

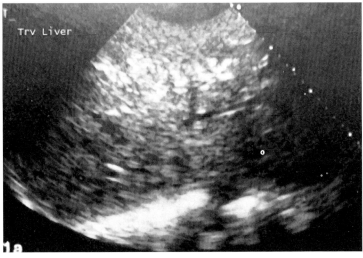

# BOWEL

## ECHOGENIC BOWEL: FOLLOW-UP IMAGING RECOMMENDED

Cystic fibrosis
Chromosomal—Trisomy 21
CMV
Intragut bleed

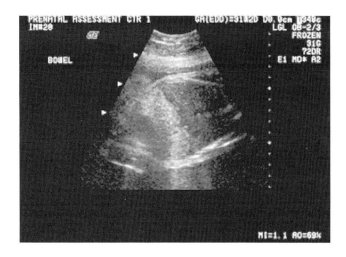

## FETAL ASCITES

### Fluids:

Blood—hemoperitoneum
Urine—collecting system
Bowel—meconium peritonitis
General—hydrops
Serous fluid—ruptured ovarian cyst

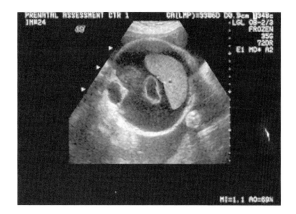

# KIDNEYS

## RENAL CYSTIC STRUCTURES

Multicystic dysplastic kidney
Severe hydronephrosis

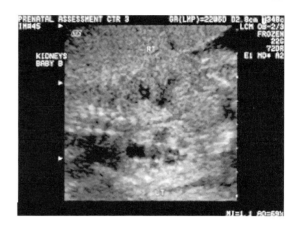

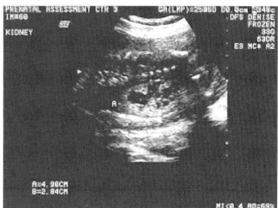

## ECHOGENIC KIDNEYS

Small—obstructive renal dysplasia

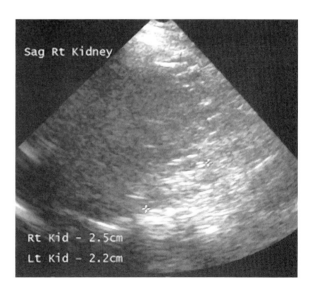

Large — APCKD, Meckel-Gruber

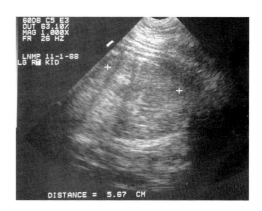

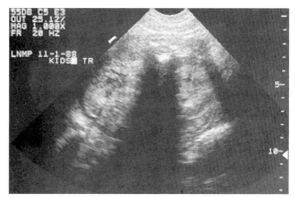

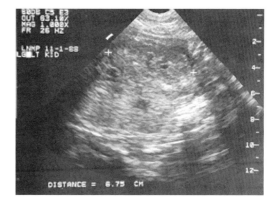

Bilateral hydronephrosis
Posterior urethral valves
Reflux
Bilateral UPJ or UVJ

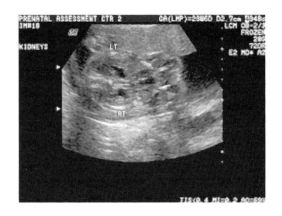

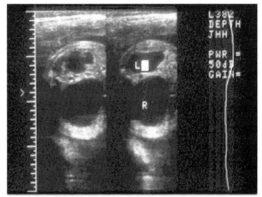

## DILATED COLLECTING SYSTEMS AND BLADDER

Obstruction, e.g., posterior urethral valves
Prune belly
Megacystitis microcolon hypoperistalsis intestinalis—polyhydramnios and intestinal obstruction

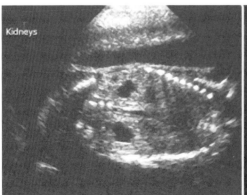
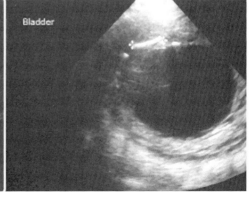

# LIMBS

## ABSENT RADIAL RAY

VATER
Trisomy 18
Fanconi's anemia
Holt-Oram syndrome—cardiac anomalies
Amniotic bands

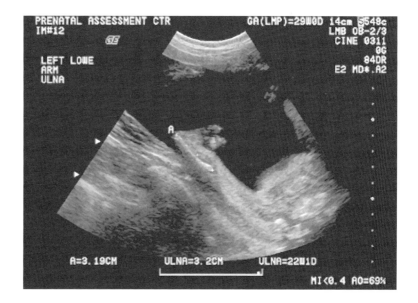

## POLYDACTYLY

Familial
Trisomy 13
Meckel Gruber—encephalocele, polycystic kidneys

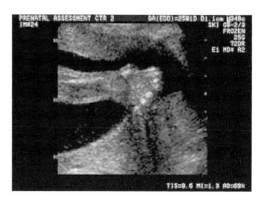

## SHORT LIMBS

Trisomy 21
Dwarfs—thanataphoric dwarf, achondrogenesis
Amniotic bands—asymmetric shortening

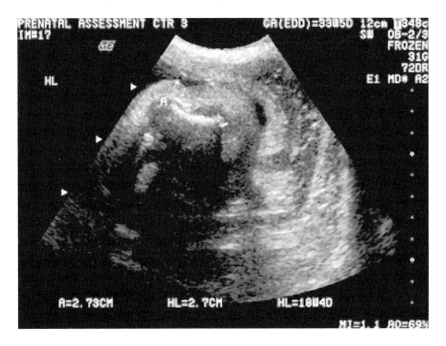

# CLUBFOOT

Idiopathic
Oligohydramnios
Trisomy 18
Amniotic bands

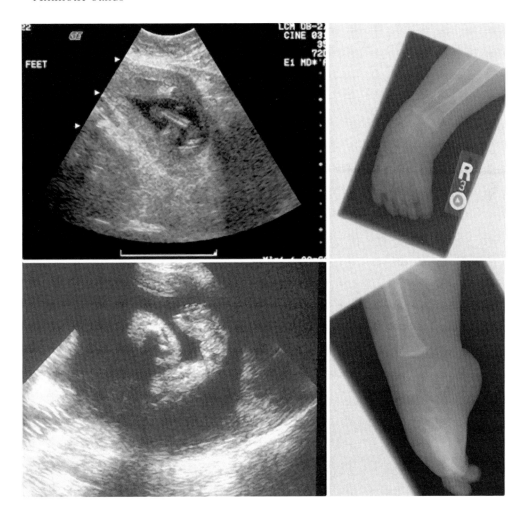

## PLACENTA + CORD

### TWO-VESSEL CORD

Renal anomalies
Cardiac anomalies
Trisomies 13 & 18

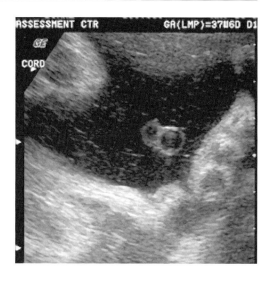

### PLACENTA AT MARGIN OF INTERNAL CERVICAL OS

Marginal previa
Full bladder
Normal until 36 wk

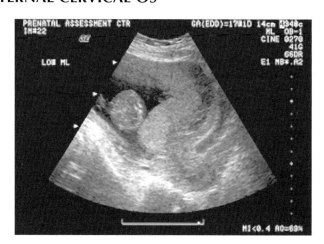

# RETROPLACENTAL COLLECTION

Placental abruption
Vascular complex
Uterine contraction
Fibroid

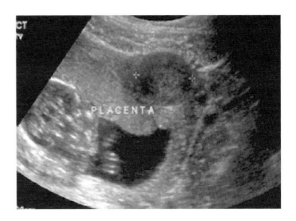

# PLACENTAL MASS

Chorangioma
Uterine contraction—NO FLOW
Fibroid—NO FLOW
Mole
Hydrops
Infection
Abruption

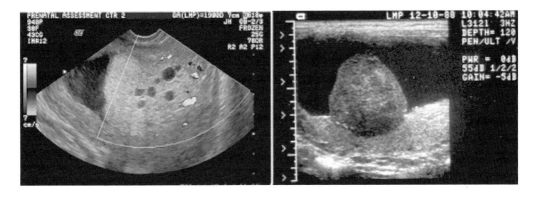

## HETEROGENEOUS MASS CONTIGUOUS WITH PLACENTA; FETUS PRESENT

Partial mole
Partial hydropic placenta
Loculated placental abruption
Chorioangioma

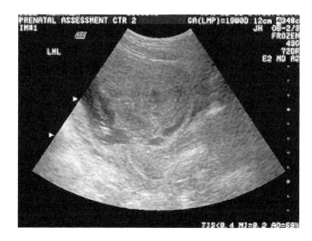
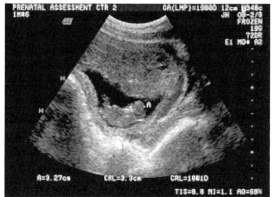

# UTERUS + OVARIES + OTHER
## MYOMETRIAL MASS DURING PREGNANCY

Uterine contraction
Fibroid
Cornual ectopic pregnancy
Extrauterine mass—adnexal, ovaries, bowel

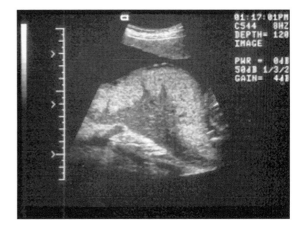

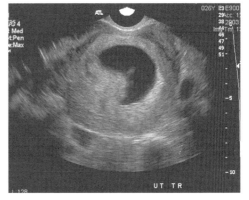

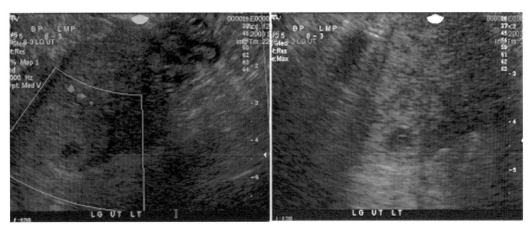

## MULTICYSTIC ENLARGED OVARY = THECA LUTEAN CYSTS

Gestational trophoblastic disease
Twins
Rh incompatibility

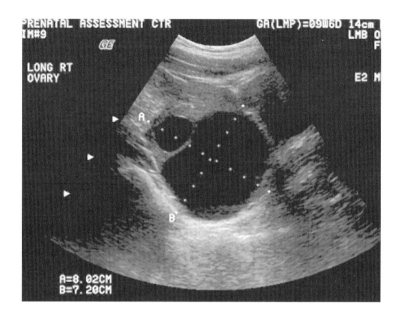

## TWO SACS IN FIRST TRIMESTER

Twins (vanishing twin)
Subchorionic hematoma
Implantation bleed
Necrotic fibroid

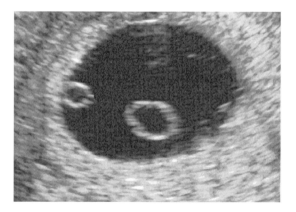

## MEMBRANE ACROSS GESTATIONAL SAC DURING SECOND AND THIRD TRIMESTER

Twins
Amniotic sheet
Circumvallate placenta

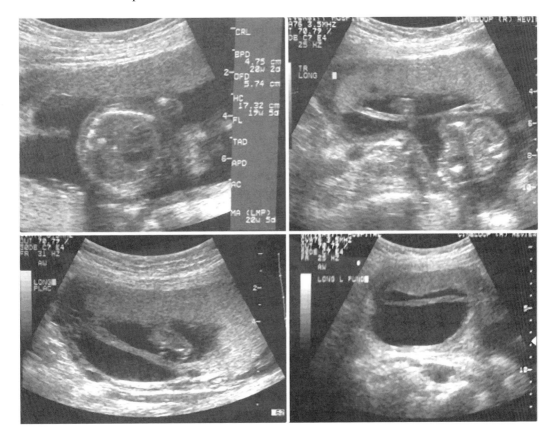

## OLIGOHYDRAMNIOS

### DRIPS

**D**emise
**R**enal
**I**UGR
**P**ROM
Po**S**tdates

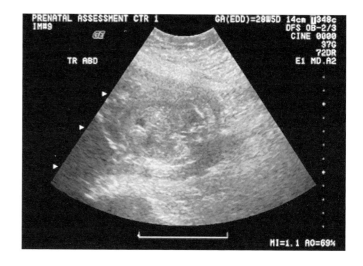

## POLYHYDRAMNIOS

### TARDI

**T**wins
**A**nomalies (fetal): esophageal atresia, duodenal/proximal small bowel obstruction, omphalocele, non-immune hydrops, anencephaly, hydranencephaly, holoprosencephaly, myelomeningocele, ventriculomegaly, agenesis of CC, encephalocele, microcephaly, diaphragmatic hernia, CCAM, tracheal atresia, extralobar sequestration, trisomy (13,18,21)
**R**h incompatibility
**I**diopathic (60%) — associated with macrosomia

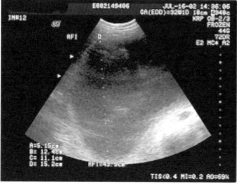
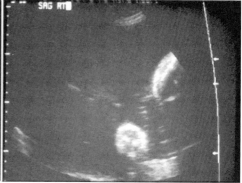

## CHROMOSOMAL ABNORMALITY SYNDROMES
### TRISOMY 13
CNS—holoprosencephaly, facial clefts
GI/GU—omphalocele, renal cystic dysplasia
MSK—polydactyly

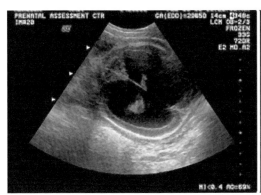
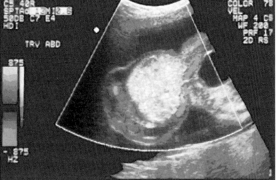
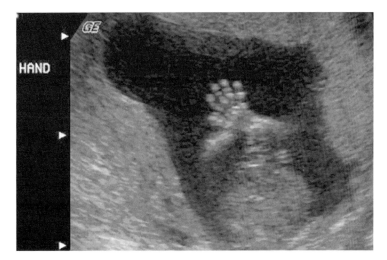

## TRISOMY 18

CNS—microcephaly, choroid plexus cysts, micrognathia, brachycephaly
GI/GU—omphalocele, diaphragmatic hernia
MSK—club foot, absent radial ray, clenched hands
Other—early symmetric IUGR, cord cyst

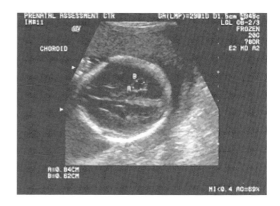

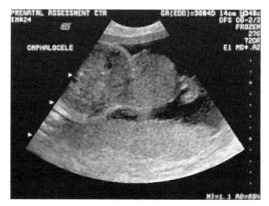

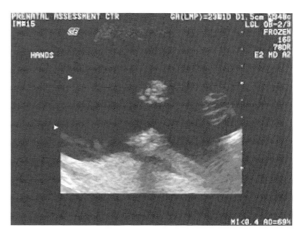

# TRISOMY 21

CNS—nuchal fold thickening, cystic hygroma
Cardiac—endocardial cushion defect, echogenic intracardiac focus
GI/GU—duodenal atresia, echogenic bowel, renal pelviectasis
MSK—short femur and humerus, widened iliac angle, clinodactyly fifth finger

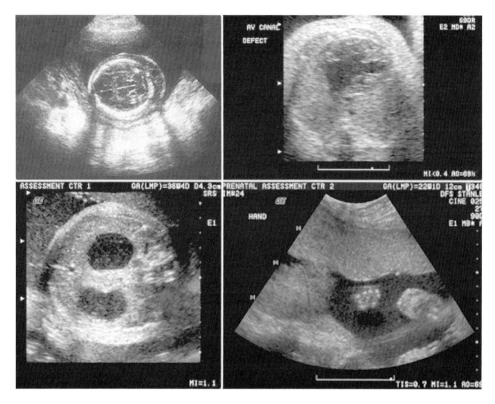
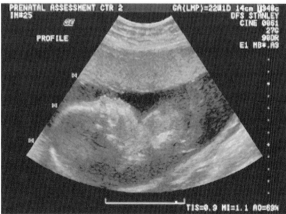

## MECKEL GRUBER

Cystic kidneys = ARPCKD
Encephalocele
Polydactyly

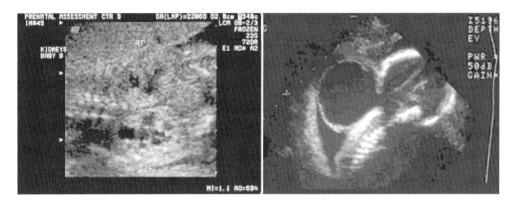

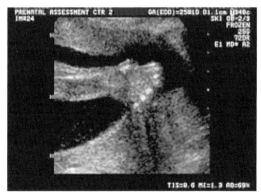

## TURNER'S

Cystic hygroma
Nuchal fold thickening
Coarctation of aorta

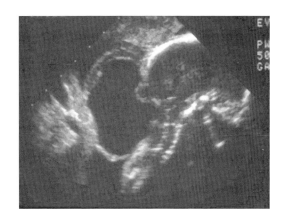
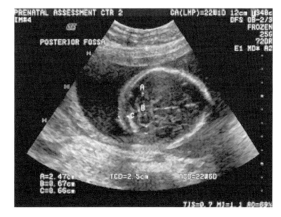
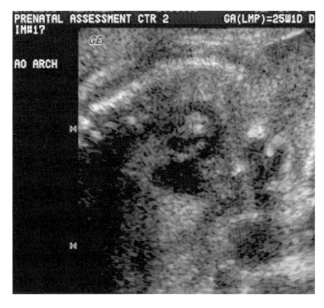

# TRIPLOIDY

Asymmetric IUGR (large head, small body)
Molar placenta

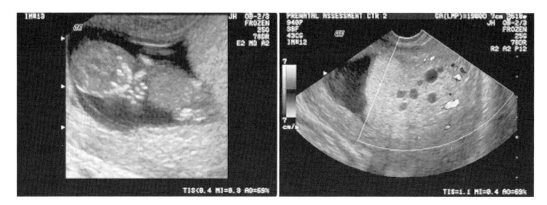

# GYNECOLOGICAL ULTRASOUND

## *Uterus*

### INTRAUTERINE COLLECTION

Retained products of conception—premenopausal
Pseudogestational sac—+βHCG
Cervical stenosis—postmenopausal
Cevical carcinoma—postmenopausal
Endometrial carcinoma—postmenopausal

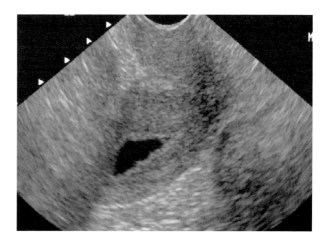

## GAS IN THE ENDOMETRIAL CAVITY

Endometritis with pyometria
Normal up to 4 wk postpartum

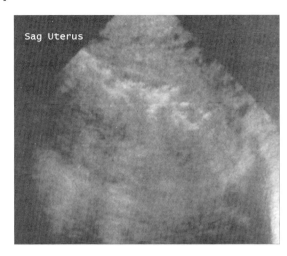

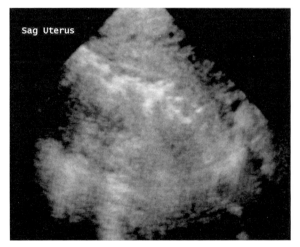

## MULTIPLE SMALL HYPOECHOIC MASSES IN THE MYOMETRIUM

Adenomyosis
Multiple fibroids

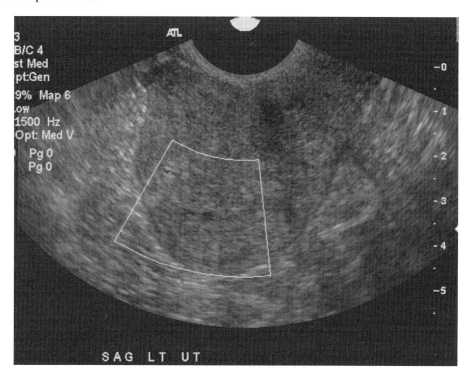

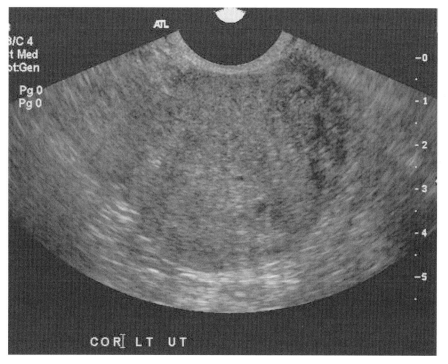

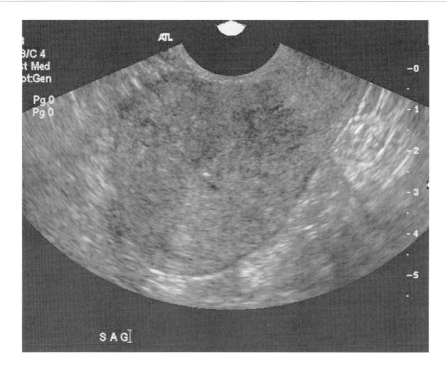

## EXTRAUTERINE COMPLEX CYSTIC MASS—DDX DEPENDS ON HISTORY, AGE, ASYMPTOMATIC, PAIN, FEVER, TRAUMA

Hemmorhagic cyst—resolve when rescan in 6 wk
Endometrioma
Teratoma
Ovarian carcinoma—more likely in postmenopausal
Ovarian torsion—pain
Tubo-ovarian abscess
Bowel abscess—appendicitis, diverticulitis
Hematoma—posttraumatic

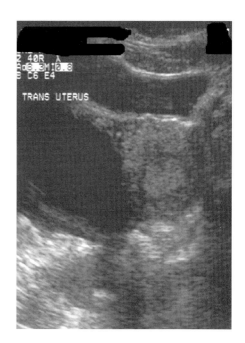

# EXTRAUTERINE SOLID MASS

Pedunculated fibroid
Endometrioma and hemmorhagic cyst
Teratoma
Ovarian torsion—pain
Fibrothecoma—ovarian
Dysgerminoma—ovarian
Ovarian metastasis, e.g., Krukenberg's tumor

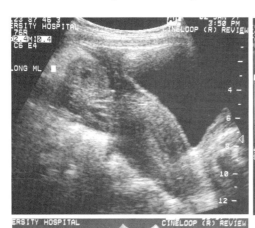
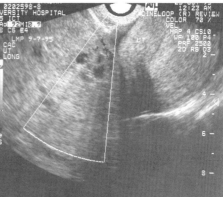
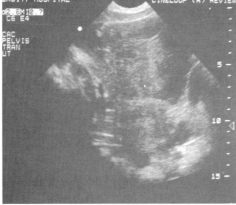

# OVARY

## OVARIAN MASS

### CHEETAH
Cyst
Hemorrhagic
Endometrioma
Epidermoid/Dermoid
Torsion
Abscess

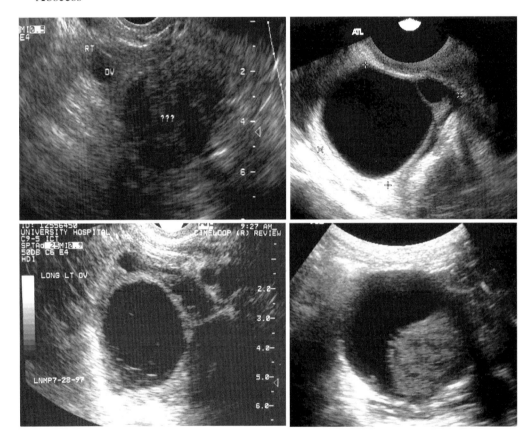

## VERY LARGE CYSTIC MASS WITH THIN SEPATATIONS

Ovarian neoplasm either benign (young) or malignant (old)
Loculated ascites—previous surgery or hemoperitoneum
Lymphangioma—previous surgery

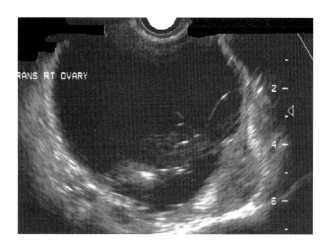

## MULTICYSTIC ENLARGED OVARY

Ovarian neoplasms—cystadenoma or cystadenocarcinoma
Ovarian torsion (pain)
Theca lutean cyst—+βHCG (bilateral)
Ovarian hyperstimulation—on Clomid (bilateral)

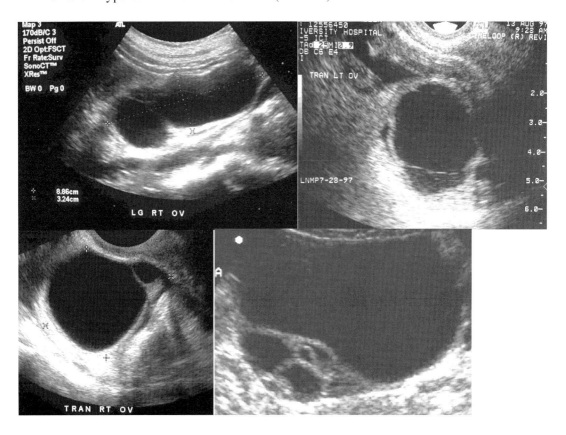

## CALCIFIED PELVIC MASS

Fibroid
Dermoid
Ovarian neoplasm

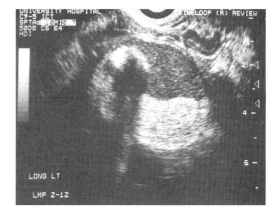

# ACUTE LOWER ABDOMEN

Torsion
Hemorrhage into ovarian cyst or endometrioma
Abscess—tuboovarian or bowel
Red degeneration of fibroid (during pregnancy)
Appendicitis

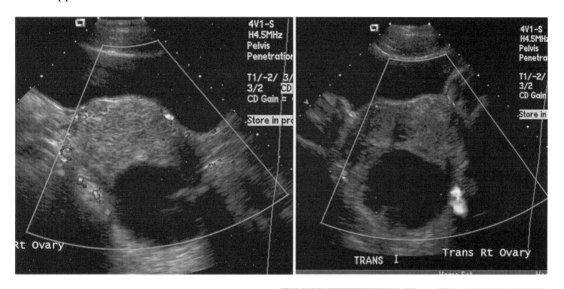

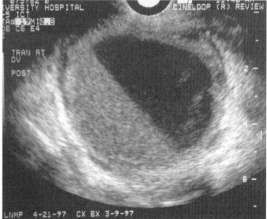

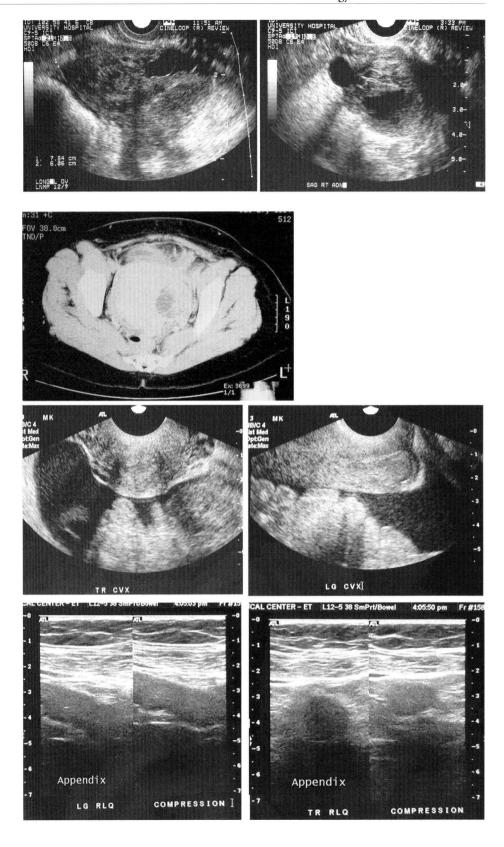

## ASCITES WITH INTRAPERITONEAL IMPLANTS

Ovarian carcinoma
Colon, pancreatic or stomach carcinoma
TB

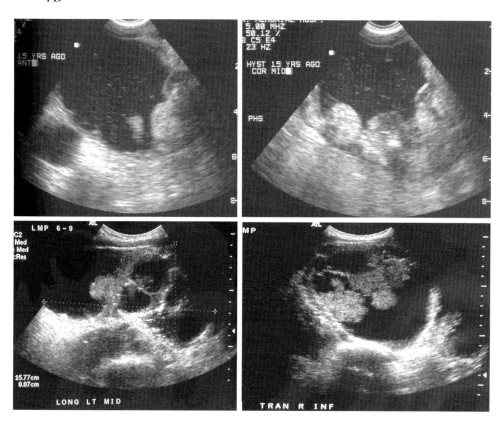

# PEDIATRIC ULTRASOUND
## CHILD WITH SOLID PELVIC MASS

Lymphoma
Malignant germ cell tumor—dysgerminoma
Sarcoma—bladder or vagina
Neuroblastoma

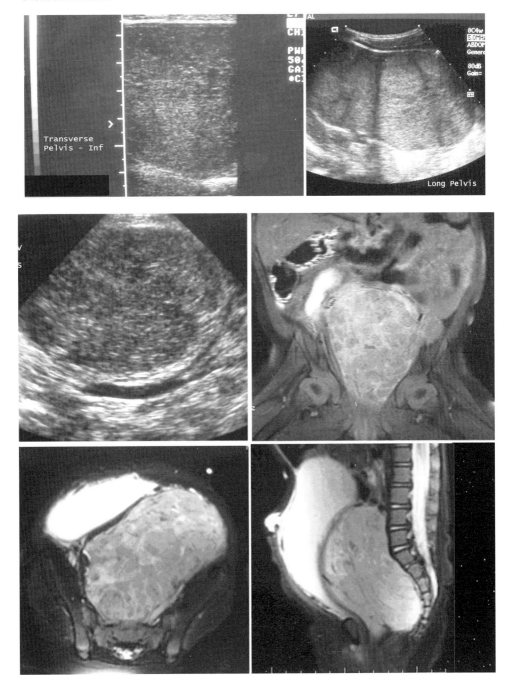

# MEDULLARY NEPHROCALCINOSIS

Lasix
Renal tubular acidosis
Tamm Horsfall proteins—rapidly resolve

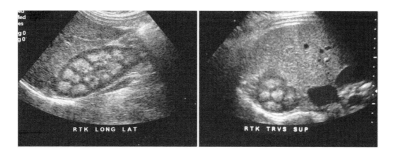

# PELVIC FLUID COLLECTION IN PREMENSES GIRL

Hematometra—cevical dysgenesis, vaginal agenesis
Hematocolpos—imperforate hymen, transverse vaginal septum

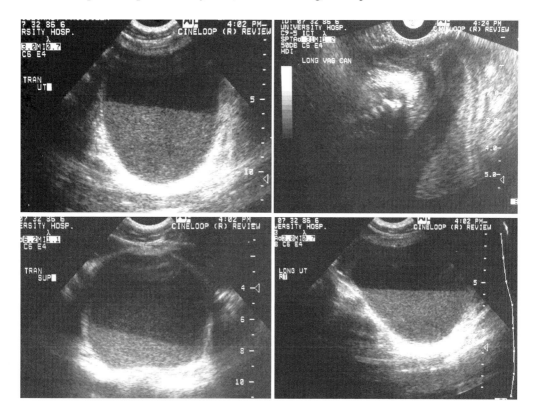

# DOPPLER ULTRASOUND

## DISCUSSIONS SHOULD INCLUDE:

1. Pulse (velocity)
2. Color (direction)
3. Power (flow)

## VARIABLES INCLUDE:

1. Doppler gain
2. Doppler scale
3. Wall filters
4. Color gain
5. Color scale
6. Color priority

# 9
# Pediatrics

*Includes imaging procedures for the diagnosis of diseases in infants and children, such as plain film radiography, contrast medium studies, ultrasound, nuclear radiology, computed tomography, digital radiography, angiography, interventional techniques, magnetic resonance imaging, and congenital heart disease.*

## Chest

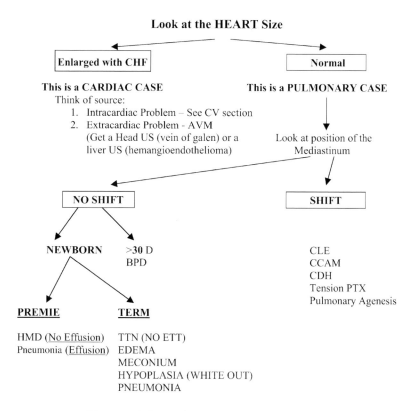

From: *Radiology: The Oral Boards Primer*
By: A. Mehta and D. P. Beall © Humana Press Inc., Totowa, NJ

EDEMA

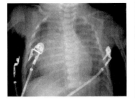 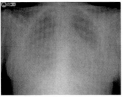

## EITHER:
### 1. CLE

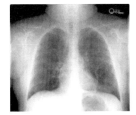 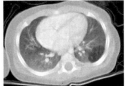 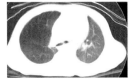

### 2. BPD

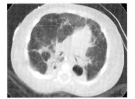 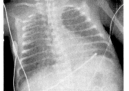

### 3. CAM

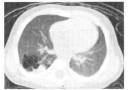 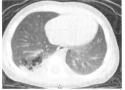

### 4. CDH

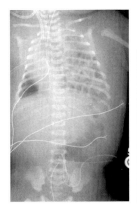 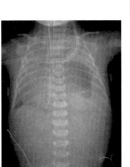 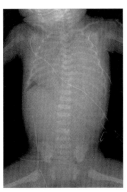

**TENSION PTX**

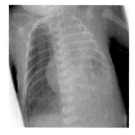 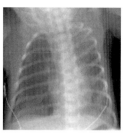

**PULMONARY AGENESIS/HYPOPLASIA WHITE OUT**

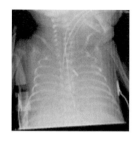

**HMD (LLV <u>NO EFF</u>)**

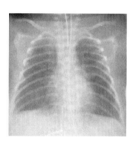

**TTN (NO ETT)**

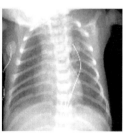 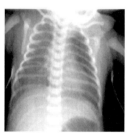 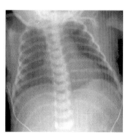

**PNEUMONIA (EFFUSION)**

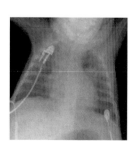

EDEMA (OBST)

MECONIUM

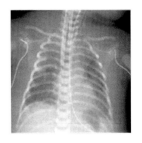

## BELL-SHAPED THORAX

Lung Hypoplasia
Abn Muscle/Bone—Dysplasia, Syndrome (JEUNE)
Nervous System—Tri 21, Paralysis

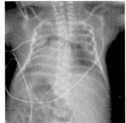 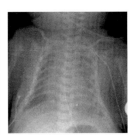

## UPPER AIRWAY

Hemangioma
Tracheitis (membranous croup)

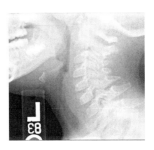

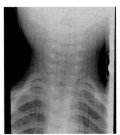

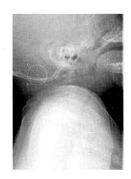

Retropharyngeal abscess

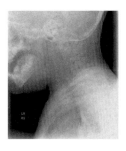

Epiglotitis

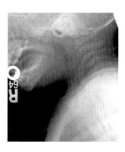

Croup

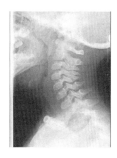

# PULMONARY MASS

## RAP'N FOREGUT

**R**ound pneumonia
**A**bscess
**P**seudotumor
**N**eoplasm (RARE) hamartoma, blastoma
**Foregut** malformations

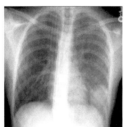 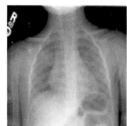 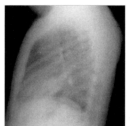 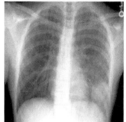

# BRONCHOPULMONARY FOREGUT MALFORMATIONS

Congenital lobar emphysema
CCAM
Sequestration
Bronchogenic cyst

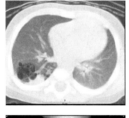 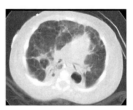 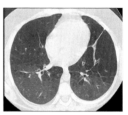
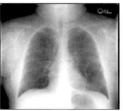 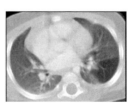 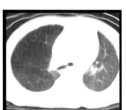

# CHEST WALL MASS
## RENAL Mets

**R**habdomyosacroma
**E**wings
**N**euroblastoma
**A**skin tumor/PNET
**L**ymphoma **Mets**

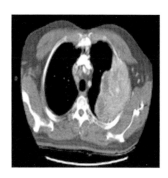

# GI/GU

## STOMACH

HPS
Spasm
Antral web

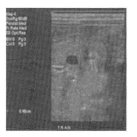
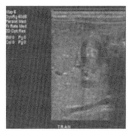
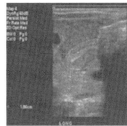
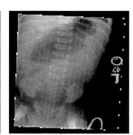

## DUODENUM

Annular pancreas
Hematoma
Preportal Duodenum
Duodenal Stenosis

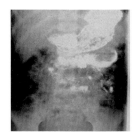
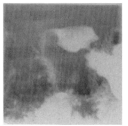
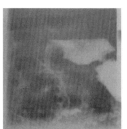

## DOUBLE BUBBLE

Duodenum
Annular pancreas
Volvulus
Ladds bands

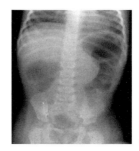
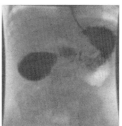

## SMALL BOWEL OBSTRUCTION
### AA II MM

Adhesion

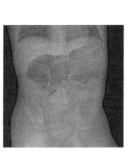
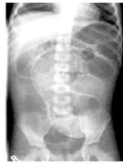
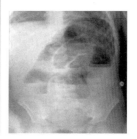

Appendicitis

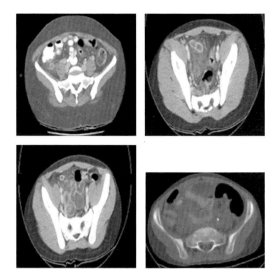

Inguinal Hernia

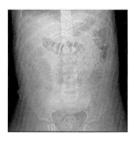

Intussusception

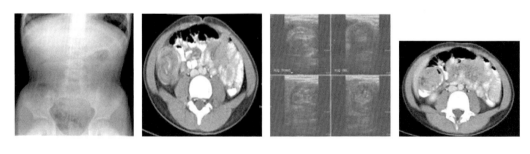

Malortation with volvulus

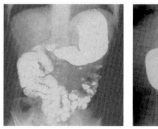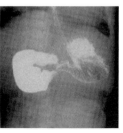

Meckels/misc

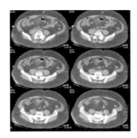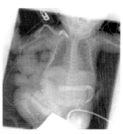

# MICROCOLON

## EVALUATE LEVEL OF DISEASE FROM LEVEL OF OBSTRUCTION:

RECTUM→SIGMOID→LEFT COLON→RIGHT COLON→TERMINAL ILEUM

Microcolon secondary to proximal atresia

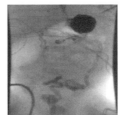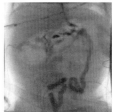

Hirschprungs (rectum)

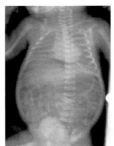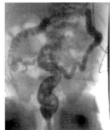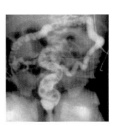

Meconium plug/Small left colon syndrome (left colon)

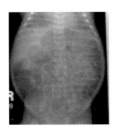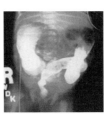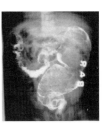

Colonic atresia (entire colon)
Ileal Atresia (entire colon)
Meconium ileus
Jejunal atresia
$MgSO_4$
Infant of a diabetic mother

# HYDRONEPHROSIS

UPJ

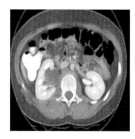 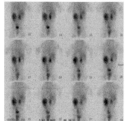

Reflux

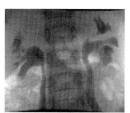 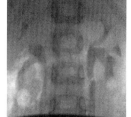

Posterior urethral valves

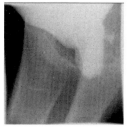 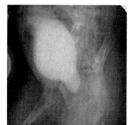

Ectopic ureterocele
Prune belly

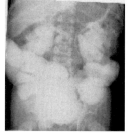 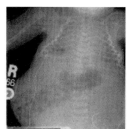

Primary megaureter
MCDK

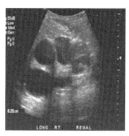 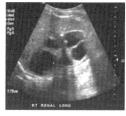

## RENAL CYSTIC DISEASE

MCDK
Juvenile nephronopthesis
APCKD
ARPCKD
Glomerulocystic disease
Obstructive lesions
NUCS CAN DIFFERENTIATE FCN/Non FCN

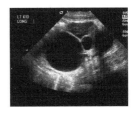

## RENAL MASS

Wilms—(chest mets) (>1 yr)

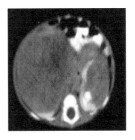

Rhabdoid—(brain mets) (1 yr)

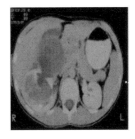

Clear cell sarcoma—(bone mets) (1 yr)
Mesoblastic nephroma

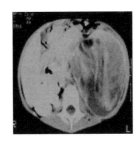 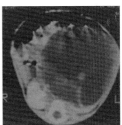

Multilocular cystic nephroma
RCC (>3 yr)
Renal medullary carcinoma (sickle cell disease)
Pyelonephritis

# BILATERAL RENAL MASSES

Nephroblastomatosis

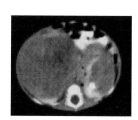 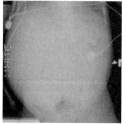

Pyelonephritis

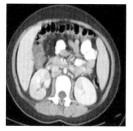 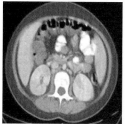

Lymphoma/mets

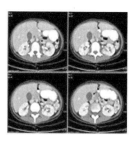 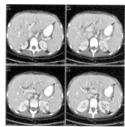

Infarcts
Cysts

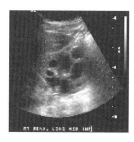 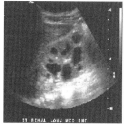

# BILATERAL ENLARGED KIDNEYS

Bilateral hydronephrosis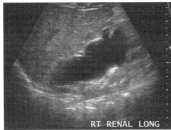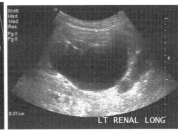

Glomerulonephritis
ARPCKD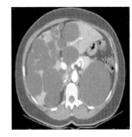

ADPCKD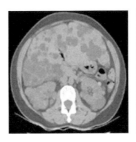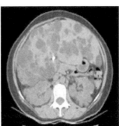

Bilateral renal vein thrombosis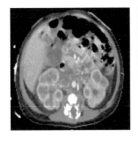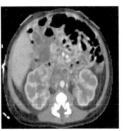

Nephroblastomatsois
Beckwith Weidemann

# ADRENAL MASS

## NAP

Neuroblastoma

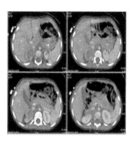 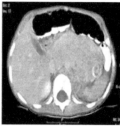 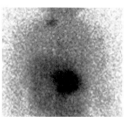 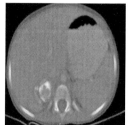

Adrenal hemorrhage/Adrenal cortical carcinoma

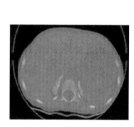 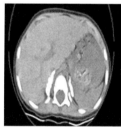 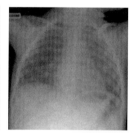

Pheochromocytoma

# BLADDER MASS
## FUR
Fibroepithelial polyp
Ureterocele

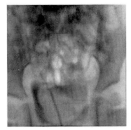 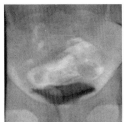

Rhabdomyosarcoma

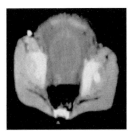 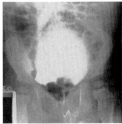 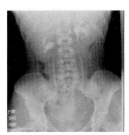

## ABDOMINAL CALCIFICATION

### L-M-N

Liver
Meconium peritonitis
Neuroblastoma

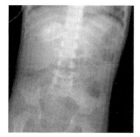 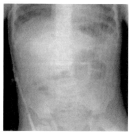

## LIVER MASS

### NEWBORN

Infantile hemangioma (solid)

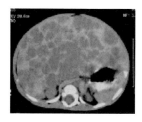

Hepatoblastoma (solid)
Embryonal cell sarcoma (mixed)

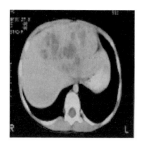

### 1 YR

Mesenchymal hamartoma (cystic)

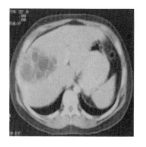

## >3 YR

Hepatocellular carcinoma (variable)

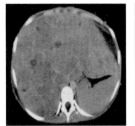 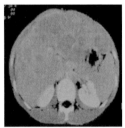

## CYSTIC ABDOMINAL MASS

### ECHO™

**E**nteric duplication
**C**holedochal cyst/mesenteric cyst
**H**ydrocolpos

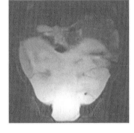 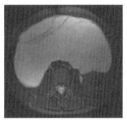

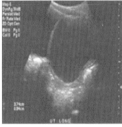 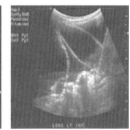

**O**varian cyst

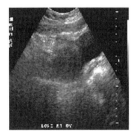 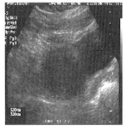

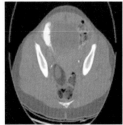

Teratoma
Meconium pseudocyst

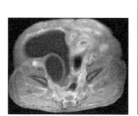
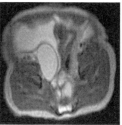

# Musculoskeletal

## MULTIPLE FRACTURES

### SHOT

Scurvy
Hypophosphatasia
OI
Trauma

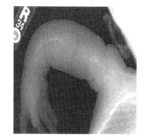

## DIFFUSE PERIOSTEAL REACTION

### SCALPR

Scurvy/infection
Caffey
Accidental trauma
Leukemia
PGE2
Rickets

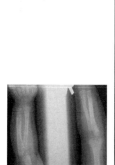 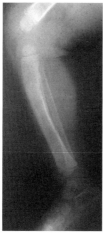 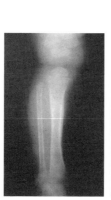 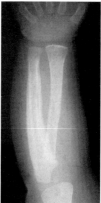 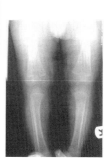

## ATLANTOAXIAL WIDENING
Downs
JRA
Morquio
Trauma

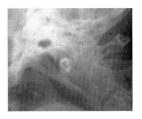

## PLATYSPONDYLY
### MODIC
Morquio
Osteogenesis imperfecta
Dwarf (thanatophoric)
Cushing's syndrome

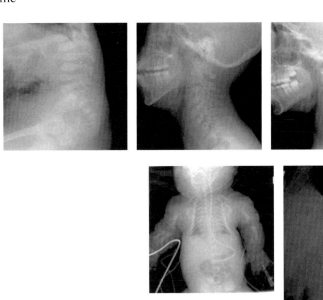

# POST VB SCALLOPING

## SALMON

**S**pinal cord tumor
**A**chondrop**L**asia
**M**ucopolysaccharidosis
**O**steogenesis imperfecta
**N**eurofibromatosis

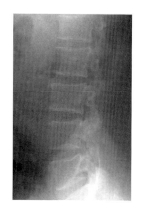

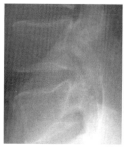

# SKULL

## 1. SCAPHOCEPHALY = DOLICOCEPHALY

Premature closure of sagittal suture (long skull)

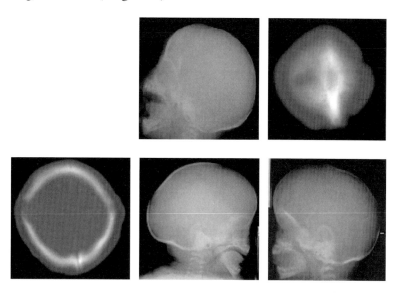

## 2. BRACHYCEPHALY = TURRICEPHALY

Premature closure of coronal/lambdoid sutures (short tall skull)

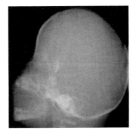 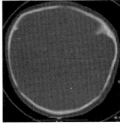

## 3. PLAGIOCEPHALY

Unilateral early fusion of coronal/lambdoidal suture (lopsided skull)

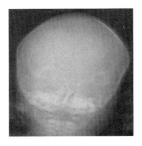

## 4. TRIGONOCEPHALY

Premature closure of metopic suture (forward pointing skull)

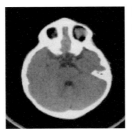 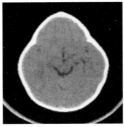 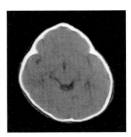

## 5. OXYCEPHALY

Premature closure of coronal, sagittal, lambdoid sutures

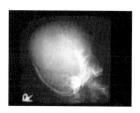

## 6. CLOVERLEAF SKULL = KLEEBLATTSCHÄDEL

Intrauterine premature closure of sagittal, coronal, lambdoid sutures

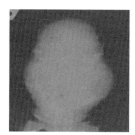 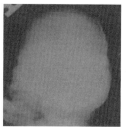

# TIBIAL BOWING

## FONAR

**F**ibrous dysplasia
**O**steogenesis imperfecta
**N**eurofibromatosis
**A**chrondroplasia
**R**ickets

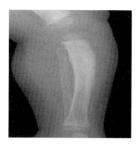

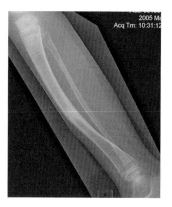

# SACRAL MASS

## KIDS WITH SACRAL MASSES **RANT**

**R**ectal duplication cyst
**A**nterior meningocele
**N**euroblastoma
**T**eratoma

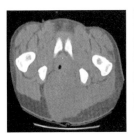 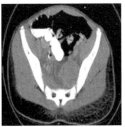 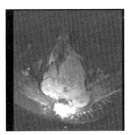

# KNEE

## POSSIBLE CASES:

Trauma
JRA
Hemophilia
TB/infection
Trevor's disease

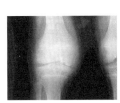 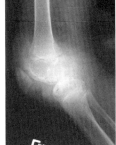 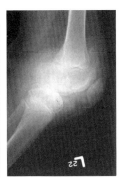

# HIP

## POSSIBLE CASES

Septic effusion
Toxic synovitis

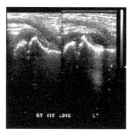 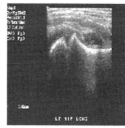 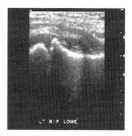

Congenital dysplasia hip (neonate/infant)

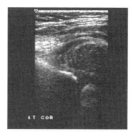 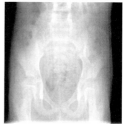

Legg Calve Perthes (school age)

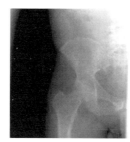 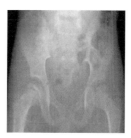

Slipped capital femoral epiphysis (adolescent)

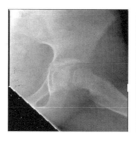 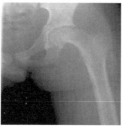 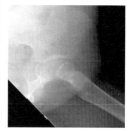

# FRAGMENTED EPIPHYSIS

## TWILL

**T**rauma
**W**arfarin
**I**nfection
**L**egg Calve Perthes
**L**eg dysplasia

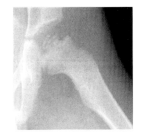

## RADIAL RAY

TAR
Holt Oram
Fanconi's anemia
Poland

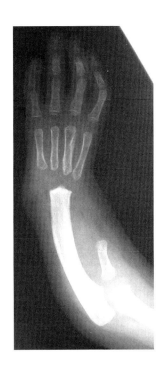

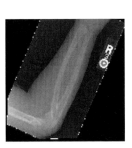
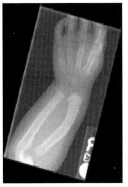

# POLYDACTYLY
Familial
Trisomy 13
Lawrence-Moon-Bardet-Biedel

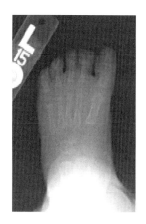

# ABUSE

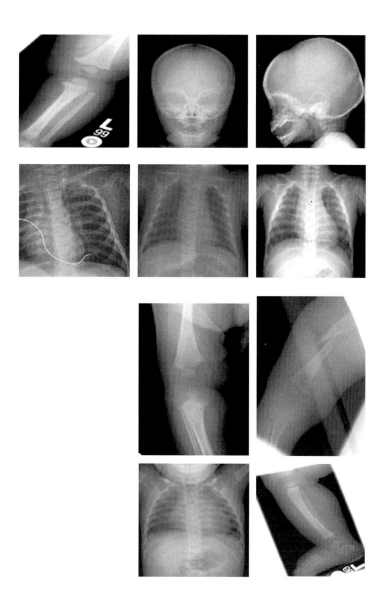

## VIEWS:

AP/LAT Axial skeleton: skull, spine, sternum
AP: Appendicular skeleton

## HIGH SPECIFICITY

Spinous process
Sternum
Scapula
Post Rib

## INTERMEDIATE SPECIFICITY

Multiple fractures in various stages of healing
Hand/wrist injury
C-Spine

## LOW SPECIFICITY

Midshaft fractures
Nonspiral fractures

# 10

# BREAST

## 1. PARENCHYMAL PATTERN ASSESSMENT
1. The breast is almost entirely fat.
2. There are scattered fibroglandular densities.
3. The breast tissue is heterogeneously dense, which may lower sensitivity of mammography.
4. The breast tissue is extremely dense, which could obscure a lesion on mammography.

## 2. MASSES ASSESSMENT
### ROLIA AND COMIS

**R**ound
**O**val
**L**obulated
**I**rregular
**A**rchitectural distortion

**C**icrumscribed
**O**bscurted
**M**icrolobulated
**I**ndistinct
**S**piculated

## 3. WORKUP NONPALP MASS
1. MAG VIEWS
2. **RO** (Round or Oval) 75% well circumscribed, not new, not bigger, not palpable
   —6 mo follow-up PB
3. Others:
   —US—CYST
   —Simple—STOP
   —Complex—ASPIRATE

From: *Radiology: The Oral Boards Primer*
By: A. Mehta and D. P. Beall © Humana Press Inc., Totowa, NJ

4. **LI** (lobulated or irregular) BX
5. **A**, Architec distortion
   —PRIOR SX? Yes—could be CA, scar, radial scar, overlap

If palp—same except US if negative mammo
Dec to bx if both negative—up to clinician

## TRABECULAR THICKENING

Inflammatory carcinoma
Mastitis
Radiation
Lymphadema/CHF

*Punch BX*

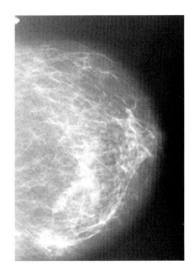

## ARCHITECTURAL DISTORTION

Carcinoma
Radial scar
Post Sx
Fat necrosis
Abscess

*? HX SURGERY*

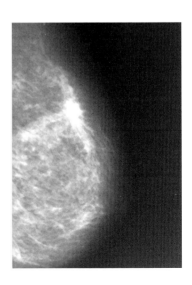

# CIRCUMSCRIBED MASS

Cyst
Fibroadenoma
Cancer
Other—phylloid/met/hematoma

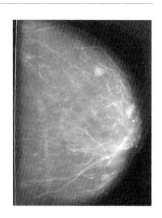

# MULTIPLE MASSES

Cysts
Fibroadenomas
Mets—melanoma/lymphoma/lung
- No HX malig 1 yr follow-up
- Hx malig

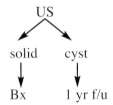

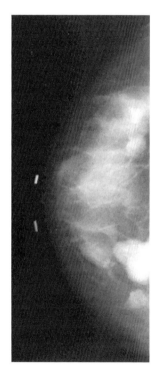

## FAT CONTAINING LESION

Hamartoma
Galactocele
Lipoma
Oil cyst

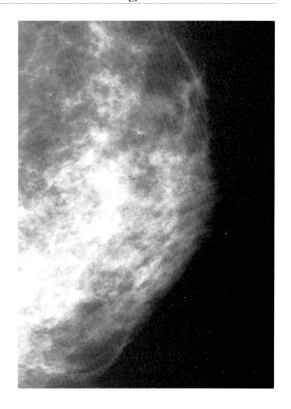

## DEVELOPING DENSITY

Carcinoma
HRT
Lymphoma
Hematoma

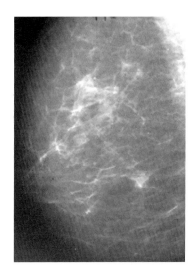
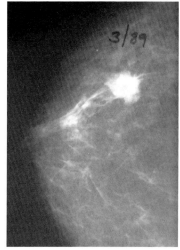

# CALCIFICATIONS

1. Identify
2. 90° VIEW to R/O MILK of calcium
3. BENIGN—STOP
   a. Vascular
   b. Popcorn
   c. Large Rods
   d. Lucent center
   e. Eggshell
   f. Suture
   g. Dystrophic

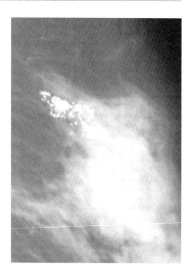

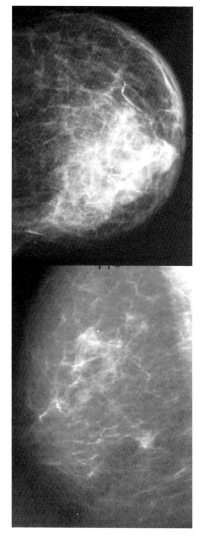

4. MALIGNANT—BX
5. Cluster round probably benign—6 mo follow-up

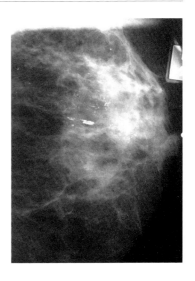

## INDETERMINATE CALCS

DCIS
Fibrocystic change, Sclerosing adenosis
Fat necrosis

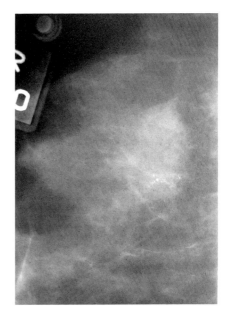

Chapter 10 / Breast

# SPECIAL

## TUBULAR DENSITY/DUCT

Nipple D/C→Serous/Bloody→US/Galactogram
Asymptomatic→STOP

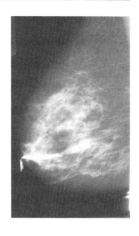

## INTRAMAMMARY LYMPH NODE

Lateral outer→Mag view fatty hilum→STOP

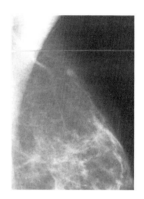

## ASYMMETRIC BREAST TISSUE

1. No calc.
2. No mass.
3. No central density.
4. No distorted architecture.

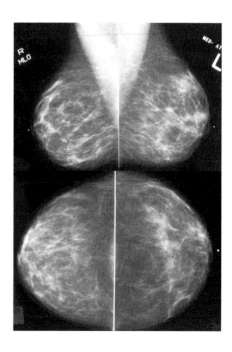

# FOCAL ASYMMETRIC DENSITY
## ? LOBULAR CARCINOMA

A. SIMILAR SHAPE ON TWO VIEWS.

B. CANNOT BE DESCRIBED WITH "ROLIA" AND "COMIS" (see p. 305)
   1. No borders, convex outward.
   2. No conspicuity of a true mass, changes on two views.
   3. Variable density.
   4. Nonpalpable.

C. MAG-ISLAND OF NORMAL BREAST TISSUE WILL RESOLVE
   If does not resolve.

D. ULTRASOUND

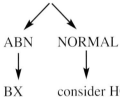

ABN    NORMAL

BX    consider HORMONE TX, If yes STOP for 3 mo. Repeat if no FOLLOW or BX (new/increasing).

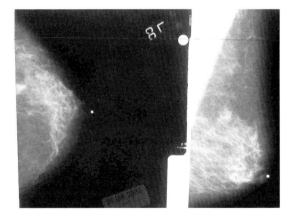

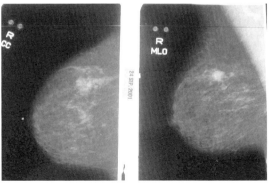

# ULTRASOUND

1. Skin
2. Superficial Fascia—Superf and Deep
   a. Fat b/w the skin and superfic
   b. Coopers b/w two layers
3. Mammary Gland
4. Retromammary Space (post to deep layer of the superficial fascia)
5. Pec Major/minor
6. Rib

# CYSTS

## SIMPLE

1. Completely anechoic
2. Smooth walls
3. Sharp ant and post borders
4. Post-acoustic enhancement

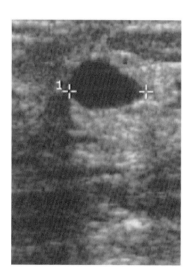

## COMPLEX

1. Abscess
2. Debris
3. Intracystic tumor (papilloma, papillary carcinoma)
4. Fat necrosis

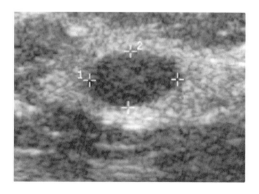

# MASSES
## THRU TRANSMIT
1. Fibroadenoma
2. Medullary carcinoma
3. Papillary carcinoma
4. Metastatic lymphoma

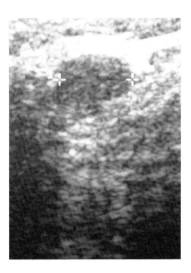

## MALIGNANT MASS

1. Spiculation
2. Taller than wide
3. Angular margins
4. Hypoechoic to fat
5. Shadow
6. Duct extension
7. Microlobulation

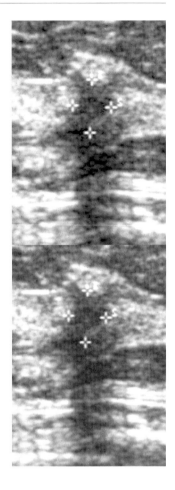

## BENIGN MASS

1. No malignant features
2. Intense, uniform echog
3. Ellipsoid plus capsule
4. Three or fewer gentle lobulations

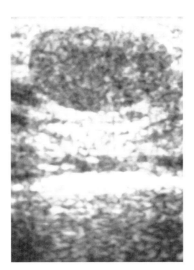
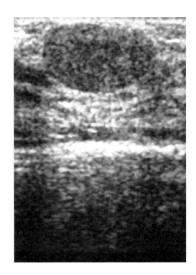

## INDETERMINATE

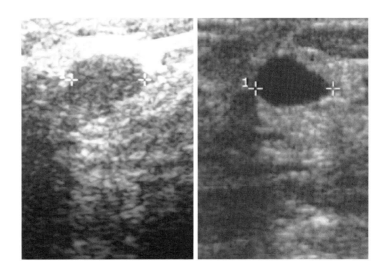

## Stereotactic Biopsies
### CONTRAINDICATIONS
1. Breast doesn't compress
2. Cant get to lesion
3. Radial Scar/Arch distortion
4. Patient cannot lie prone

# 11
# Neuroradiology

*Includes plain film diagnosis of the skull, sinuses, mastoids, spine and head, and neck structures, and all other imaging and special procedures related to the central nervous system and head and neck including angiography, myelography, interventional techniques, and magnetic resonance imaging.*

## IN GENERAL, EVERY CASE WILL FALL INTO:
1. Tumor
2. Infarct (arterial or venous)
3. Infection
4. Vascular
5. Congenital
6. Inflammatory

## EVERY CASE TO PREVENT FAILING THE SECTION:
1. IS IT VASCULAR?
2. IS THERE HERNIATION?

From: *Radiology: The Oral Boards Primer*
By: A. Mehta and D. P. Beall © Humana Press Inc., Totowa, NJ

# White Matter

## DEMYELINATING

### *Cortical*

#### LATE VIDEO

**L**ymphoma
**A**DEM
**T**rauma
**E**lderly-nonspecific periventricular
**V**asculitis
**I**nfections HIV/Herpes/PML
**D**emyelinating
**E**clampsia
**O**ther—Radiation Tx

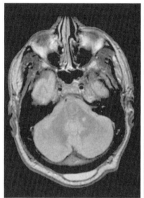
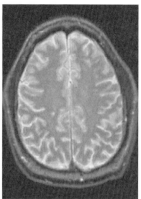
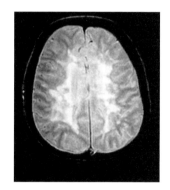
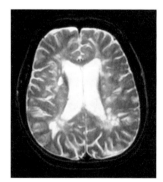
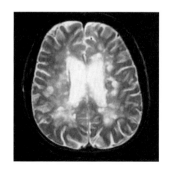

## Brainstem

### Central Pontine Myelinolysis

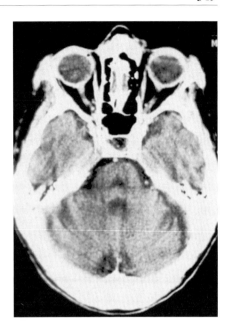

# DYSMYELINATING

## LACK OF Proper Myelination

Leigh (Leigh's **PUT**ATO chips)
 —**Put**amen, periventricular, subcortical
**A**drenoleukodsytrophy—Posterior
**A**lexander—Big head, Frontal
**C**anavan—Big Head, Subcortical
**K**rabbe—Thalami
**P**elizeus Merzbacher—Diffuse
**M**etachromic Leuko—Cerebellar+BG

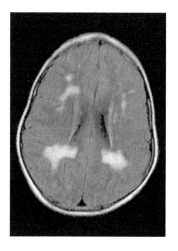

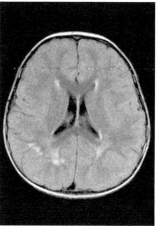

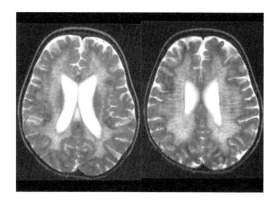

# ATROPHY

## CORTICAL

Senile dementia Alzheimer's type
Ischemic/Vascular
Picks

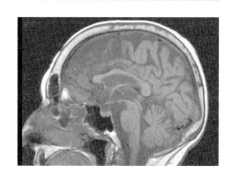

## BASAL GANGLIA/OTHER

Parkinson's

# MULTIPLE MASSES

## MAILMAN

**M**etastasis
**A**ngiomas — Vascular malformations
**I**nfarction/infection
**L**ymphoma
**M**ultiple sclerosis
**A**bscesses
**N**F spots (remember the esoteric diagnoses)

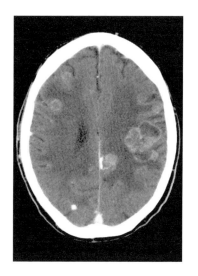

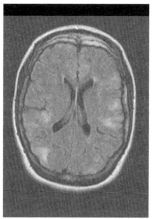

# EXTRA AXIAL MASS

## MAD SALE

Mengioma
Abscess
Dural metastasis—prostate/breast

Sarcoidosis
Abscess/AVM
Lymphoma
Epidermoid/dermoid

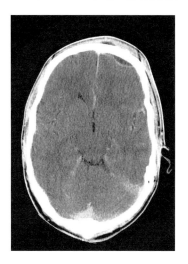

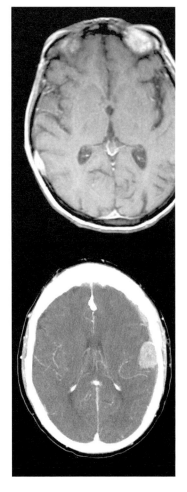

## INTRA-AXIAL

*Supratentorial*

### CHILD

#### TAPE

    Teratoma
    Astrocytoma
    PNET
    Ependymoma

### ADULT

#### WHITE MATTER

##### OLD MAN

    Oligodendroglioma
    Lymphoma
    Dermoid

    Metastasis
    Astrocytoma
    Neuronal tumors

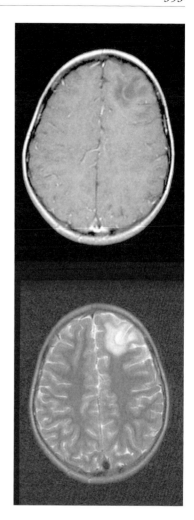

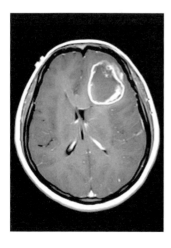

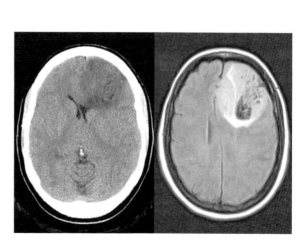

# INFECTION

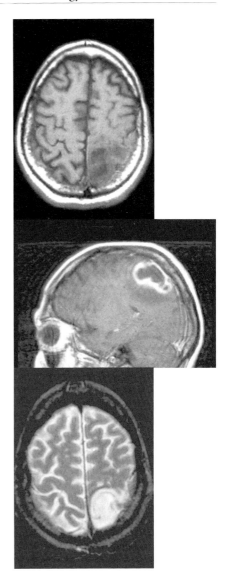

# CORTICAL

## TIGER TIM

**T**rauma
**I**nfarct
**G**angliogioma/glioma
**E**ncephalitis
**R**adiation

**T**ubers
**I**nfection—toxoplasmosis
**M**etastasis

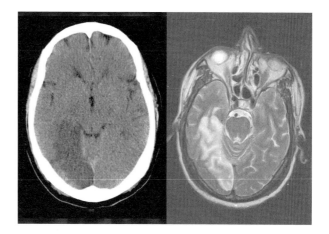

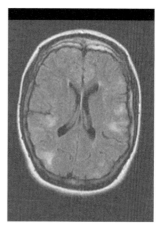

## Infratentorial

### CHILD

*Cerebellum*

Medulloblastoma—(precontrast hyperintense)
Ependymoma—($Ca^{2+}$)(cystic)
JPA
Mets
Choroid plexus papilloma

*Brainstem*

Brainstem glioma+tectal glioma

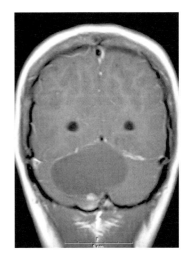

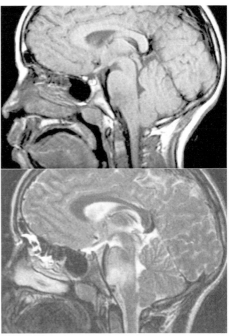

# Adult

*Cerebellum*

Mets
Hemangioblastoma
Astrocytoma
Choroid plexus C/P
Lymphoma

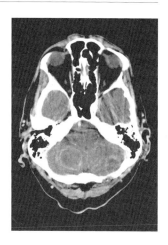

*Brainstem*

**Tumor**
Metastasis
Brainstem Glioma

**Infection**
Tb
Abscess

**Inflammatory/Vascular**
Cavernoma/AVM
Infarct

**Demyelinating**

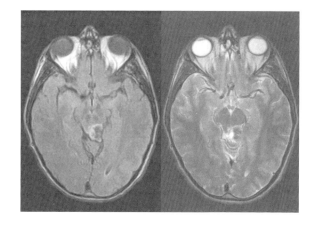

## TEMPORAL LOBE

Tumor: Ganglioglioma
Infection: Herpes
Vascular: Transverse sinus
   thrombosis/infarct

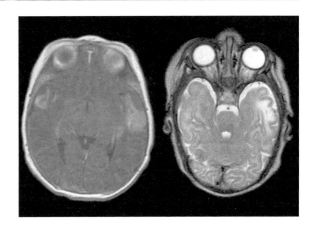

## CALCIFIED TUMORS

### OLD ELEPHANTS AGE GRACEFULLY AND LIKE PEANUTS

**O**ligo
**E**pendymoma
**A**strocytoma
**G**BM
**P**NET

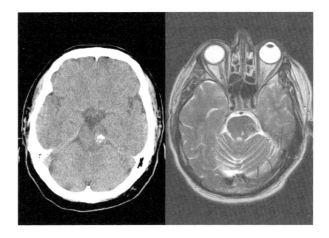

# SELLAR

## PC OR MAC?

**P**ituitary adenoma/apoplexy
**C**raniopharyngioma
**M**ets/meningioma
**A**bscess/Aneurysm
**C**ysts—Rathke's cleft

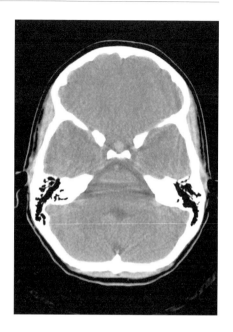

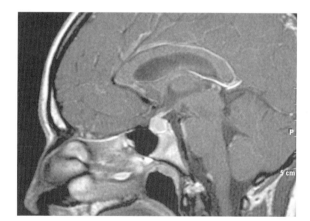

# SUPRASELLAR
## SATCHMOE

Sarcoid
Aneurysm
Teratoma/germinoma
Craniopharyngioma
Hamartoma of the tuber cinereum
Meningioma/mets
Optic glioma
EG

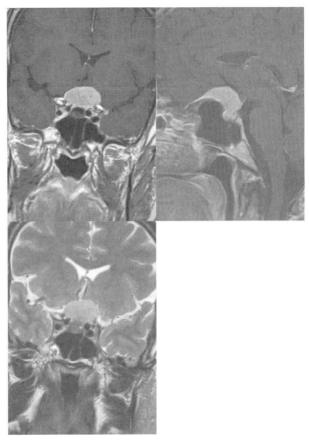

# PARASELLAR MASS
## MCAT

Meningioma/metastasis
Cavernous carotid fistula
Aneurysm
Trigeminal Schwannoma/Tolosa-Hunt

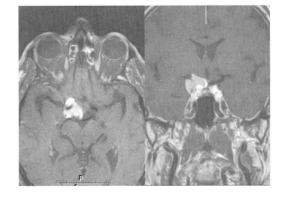

# INFUNDIBULAR MASS

## MEET GIRLS

Metastasis
Eosinophillic granuloma
Germinoma/germ cell tumors
Infection/inflammation (hypophysitis)
DuRal–(think of dural-based conditions)
Lymphoma
Sarcoid

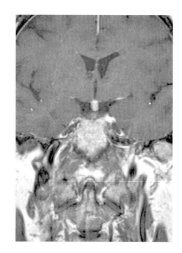

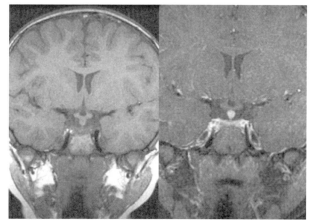

# PINEAL MASS

## MAD PIG

**M**eningioma/metastasis
**A**rachnoid cyst/Aneurysm/AVM
**D**ermoid/teratoma

**P**ineal parenchymal tumor
**PI**neal cyst
**G**erm cell tumor/Glioma

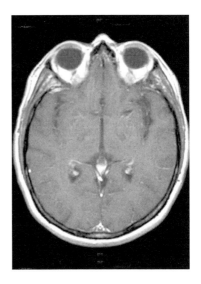

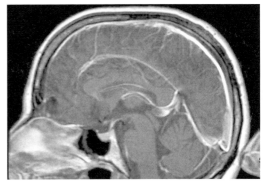

# CP ANGLE

## SLow GAME

Schwanomma: V and VII
Lymphoma/lipoma
Glomus tumor
Aneurysm
Meningioma/Metastasis
Epidermoid/Ependymoma

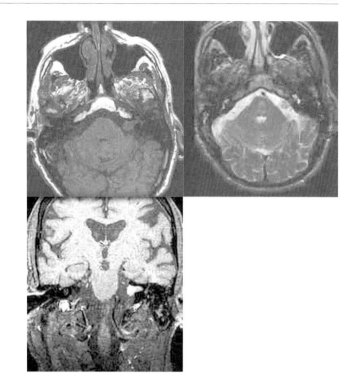

# Ventricular Disorders

## VENTRICULITIS

**Infection**—CMV/HIV/TB

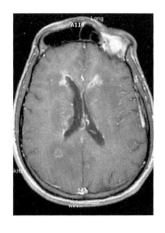

**Tumor**—Carcinoma/metastasis/lymphoma

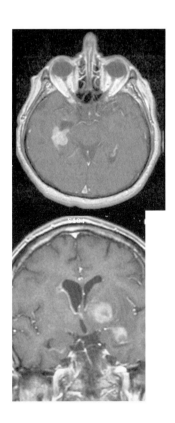

# MASS

## Adult

### EMC[2]

**E**pendymoma/Gliomas
**M**ets/Meningioma
**C**horoid plexus tumors
**C**entral neurocytoma/Cystercercosis

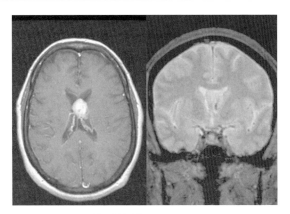

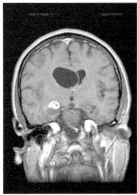

## Child

### PETA (save animals)

**P**NET
**E**pendymoma
**T**eratoma
**A**strocytoma

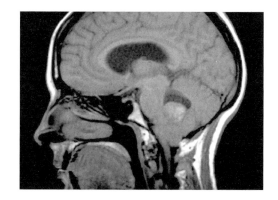

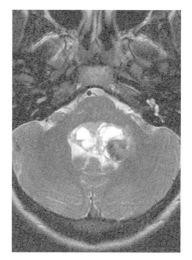

# HYDROCEPHALUS

## *Communicating*
NPH (wet, wobbly, wacky)
Meningitis
Post subarachnoid hemorrhage
Post surgery

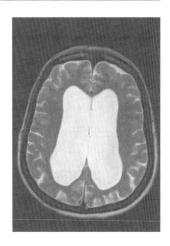

## Noncommunicating
- 3rd ventricular mass
- Aqueductal tumors/stenosis
- 4th ventricular mass

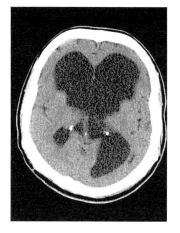

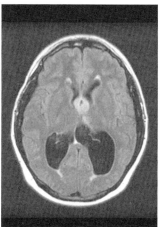

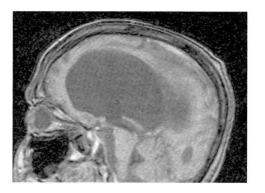

# INFARCTS/STROKE

1. Large vessel—MCA/ACA/PCA

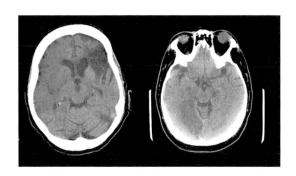

2. Watershed

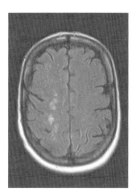

3. Small vessel disease—Lacunes. HTN

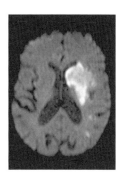

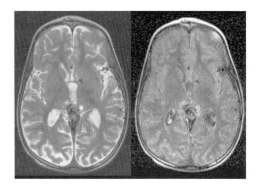

4. Microvascular—Leukariasis

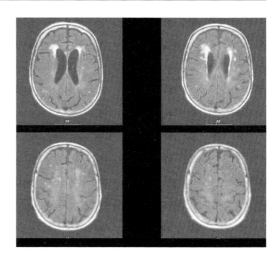

5. Posterior fossa (may need to be decompressed)

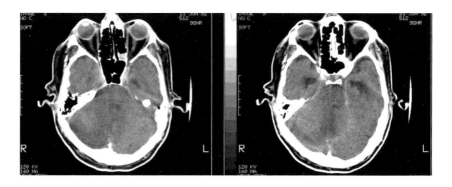

## ARTERIAL CAUSES

Thrombosis/atherosclerosis
   —Check Circle of Willis/branch points
Dissection—Check neck vessels
Low flow—Check history
Emboli-Drug history
Vasculitis

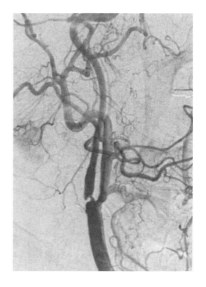

## VENOUS CAUSES
### SHIPPED

**S**ickle cell
**H**ypercoaguable
**I**nfarct
**I**nfection
**P**regnancy
**P**ill (oral contraceptives)
**E**ndogenous—Factor V Leiden
**D**ehydration

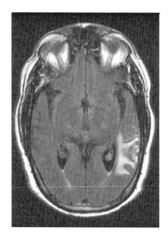

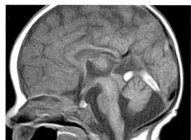

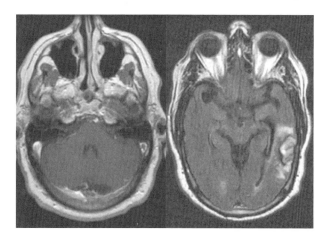

# INTRAPARENCHYMAL HEMATOMA

## Young

### DATA

**D**rug abuse—Cocaine
**A**neurysm
**T**umor—Underlying
**A**VM/Vascular malformations

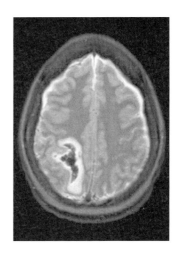

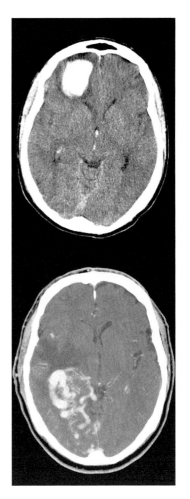

## Old

### HAT

**H**TN—putamen/thalamus/pons/cerebellum
**A**myloid/Anticoagulation
**T**umor—primary or metastasis

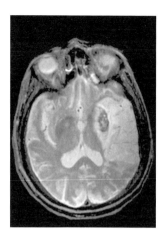

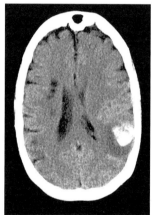

# RING-ENHANCING LESION

## MAGIC DR

### Immunocompromised
Toxoplasmosis vs lymphoma

### Immunocompetent
**M**ets
**A**bscess
**G**lioma
**I**nfarct
**C**ontusion

**D**emyleinating (MS)
**R**adiation Necrosis

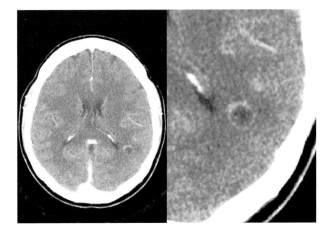

# CROSSING LESIONS OF THE CORPUS CALLOSUM

Lymphoma
GBM
MS
ADEM/PML
Trauma
Metastases

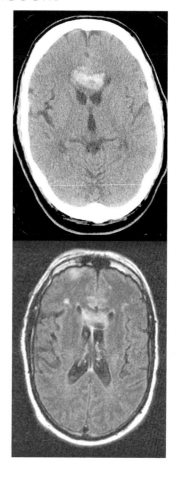

## LEPTOMENINGEAL ENHANCEMENT

Carcinomatosis—breast/lung/melanoma
Infection—viral or bacterial meningitis/TB
Inflammatory—sarcoid
Consider subarachnoid hemorrhage
Spontaneous intracranial hypotension

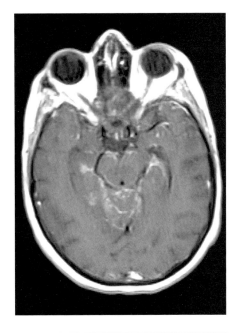

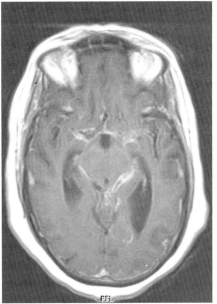

# DURAL ENHANCEMENT

Postoperative
Spontaneous intracranial hypotension
Metastatic disease—breast/prostate
Sarcoidosis

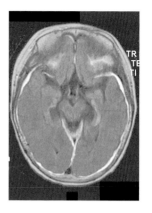

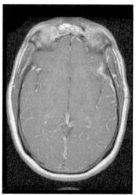

# CONGENITAL

## Children Complete Myelination at 2 yr of Age

### DISORDERS OF NEURAL TUBE CLOSURE

Cephalocele

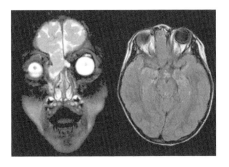

Corpus Callosal anomaly—Agenesis

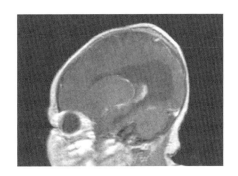

Dandy Walker malformation

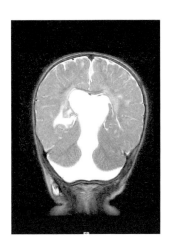

Chiari II
Migrational disease

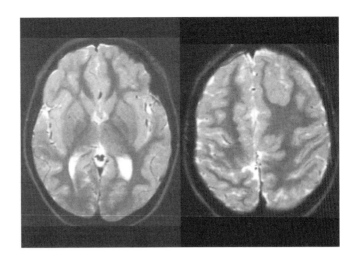

Idiopathic
Lipomas

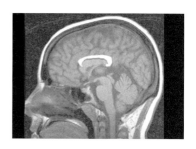

Cysts—Aicardi's syndrome
Hydranencephaly
Porencephaly—toxoplasmosis

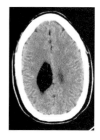

Dyke Davidoff Mason—unilateral atrophy

## Disorders of Neuronal Migration

Lissencephaly
Nonlissencephalic cortical dysplasia
  *ASSOCIATED WITH CMV—affinity for germinal matrix*

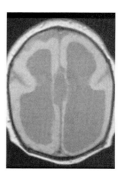

Heterotopia

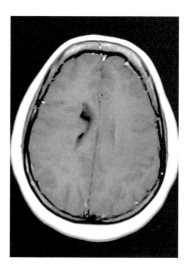

## Chapter 11 / Neuroradiology

Schizencephaly

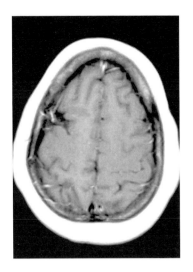

Unilateral megalencepahly

### DISORDERS OF DIVERTICULATION
Holoprosencephaly

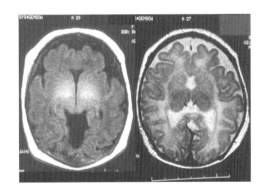

Septo-optic dysplasia

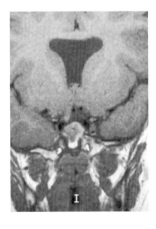

Absence of SP— *LOOK FOR SEPTO-OPTIC AND SCHIZENCEPHALY*

# Cystic Posterior Fossa
DW Complex

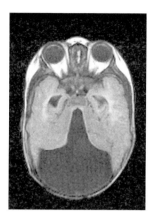

DW Variant
MCM
Arachnoid Cyst

# Cerebral Angiography

Angiograms shown in the Neuro section will be looking for specific diagnoses based on the region in which they are shown. These are:

## ANGIOGRAPHIC DDX

### AORTIC ARCH

*Vessel Irregularity*

Atherosclerosis

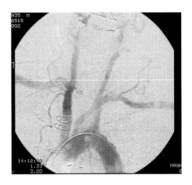

Vasculitis

Trauma

# EXTERNAL CAROTID ARTERY

*Tumor*

Meningioma
Juvenile Angio

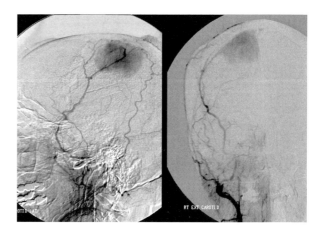

Chemodectoma

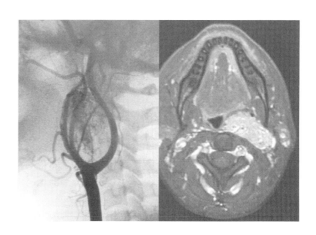

# CERVICAL CCA/ICA/VERT

*Vessel Irregularity*

Atherosclerosis

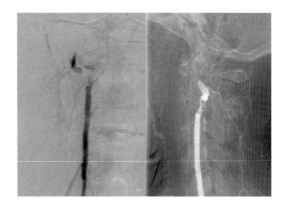

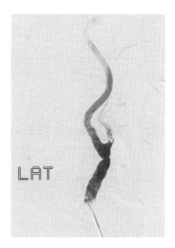

FMD
Dissection
Trauma

*Neoplasm*

Paraganglioma

*AVM—Dural-based*

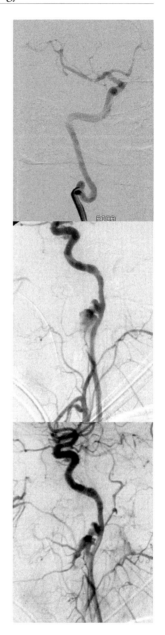

## PETROUS INTERNAL CAROTID ARTERY
Trauma

Aneurysm

## INTRACRANIAL ICA

Aneursym

CCF

Occlusion

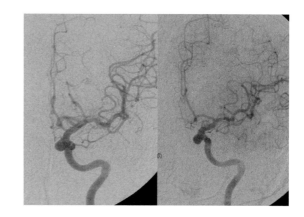

## CIRCLE OF WILLIS

Aneurysm

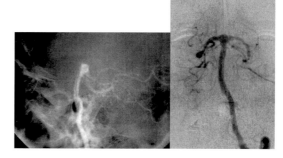

AVM

Stenosis

Tumor
    Meningioma
    Hemangioblastoma

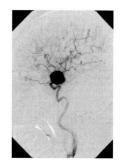

# INTRACRANIAL

## VASCULAR MALFORMATIONS

AVM—parenchymal/dural/cryptic

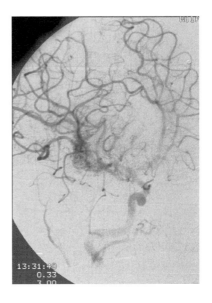

Venous angioma (deep venous anomaly)/cavernoma

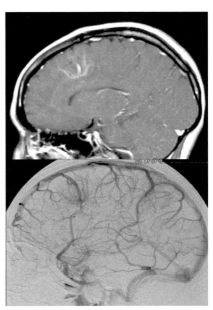

# Cavernous Angioma

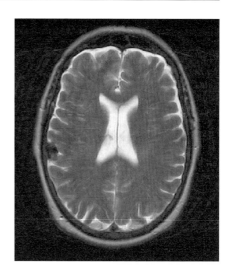

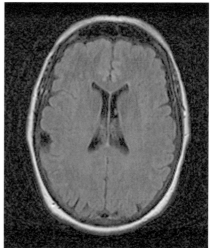

## Capillary Telangiectasia

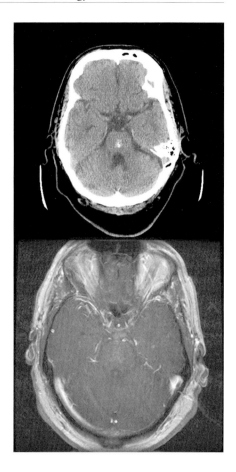

# VASCULITIS

| *Infectious* | *Noninfectious* | *Atypical* | *Nondrug* |
|---|---|---|---|
| TB | Cocaine | Drug ergots | Sarcoid |
| Syphillis | Amphetamine | | Wegener's |
| | | | PAN |

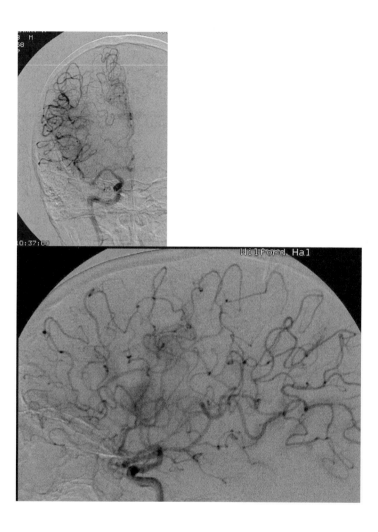

## CHILDREN/INFANTS

Moya Moya
NF
Sickle
Radiation
Idiopathic
Vein of Galen malformation

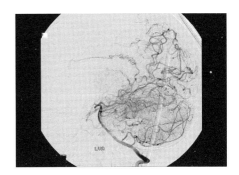
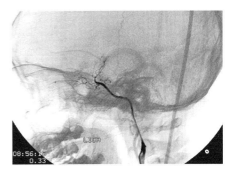
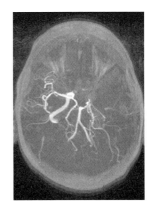

# CSF SEEDING

## PAGE ME

**P**apillomas—choroid plexus/carcinoma
**A**strocytomas—GBM
**G**erminoma
**E**pendymoma
**ME**dulloblastoma

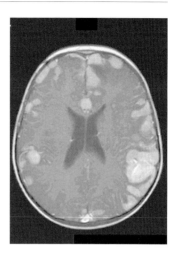

# BASAL GANGLIA CA$^{2+}$ HYPERDENSE ON CT/HYPOINTENSE ON T1

## BIRTH

**B**irth Anoxia
**I**nfection—HIV
**R**adiation
**T**oxin—Carbon Monoxide/Lead/TPN
**H**ypoparathyroidism/Hypophosphatasia

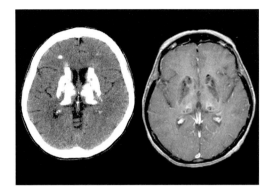

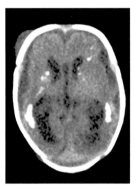

# BASAL GANGLIA DISEASES HYPODENSE ON CT/HYPERINTENSE ON T2

## LINT

**L**ymphoma
**I**nfarction—hypoxia/hypotension
**N**eurodegenerative—Wilson's
**T**oxins—Carbon Monoxide/Cyanide/Choloroethane

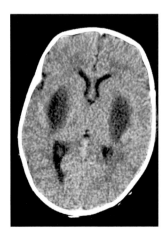

# DIFFUSE CEREBRAL EDEMA

## HIGH PRESSURE

**H**ypertensive crisis
**P**seudotumor
**R**eye's syndrome
**E**ncephalitis
**S**agittal **S**in**U**s th**R**ombosis
**E**clampsia

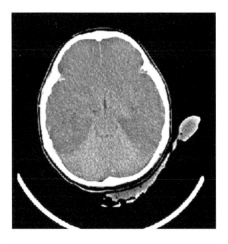

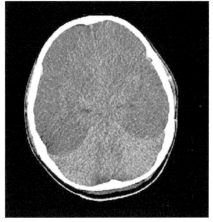

# SPECTROSCOPY

Normal Spectrum

```
                        x
                        x
                        x
     x   x              x        x
     x   x              x        x
    xxxxx  xxxxxxxxxxx xxxxxx xxxxxxx
    Choline  Creatine   NAA    Lactate
```

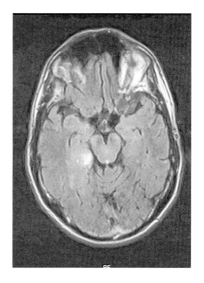

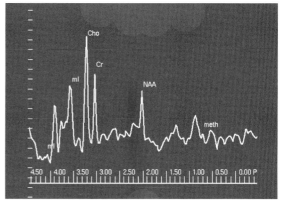

Rules of Thumb

1. Low grade tumor and demyelination can look identical.
2. Very high choline levels usually indicates tumor.
3. Infarct shows elevated lactate and decreased other values.
4. Increased lactate in the CSF can be seen in NPH.
5. Decreased NAA indicates neuronal loss
   (including neuronal loss seen in tumor).

# Spine

## INTRADURAL INTRAMEDULLARY

### AHEM, MIGHT I help you?

**A**strocytoma
**H**emangioblastoma
**E**pendymoma
**M**ets

**M**S
**I**nfection/myelitis
**G**ranulomatous – sarcoid
**H**emorrhage
**T**rauma

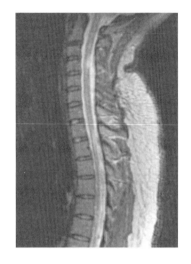

## INTRADURAL EXTRAMEDULLARY

### DAMN VASCULAR HEMATOMA

**D**ural mets
**A**VM/arachnoid cyst
**M**eningioma
**N**F/Schwanomma

**V**ascular

**H**ematoma

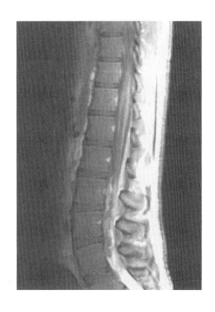

# EXTRADURAL EXTRAMEDULLARY

## SMALL HEAD

**S**ynovial cyst
**M**ets/Meningioma/Schwanomma
**A**VM
**L**ymphoma
**L**eukemia

**H**ematoma
**E**pidural Abscess
**A**denopathy
**D**isk
   Bulge
   Herniation—Extrusion/Protrusion
   Free Fragment

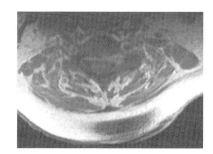

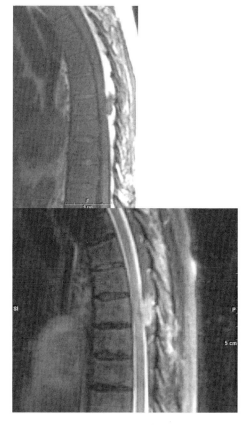

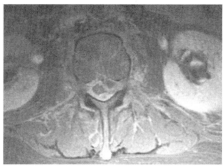

# ARACHNOIDITIS

Failed back syndrome
Subarachnoid hemorrhage
Infection
Pantopaque

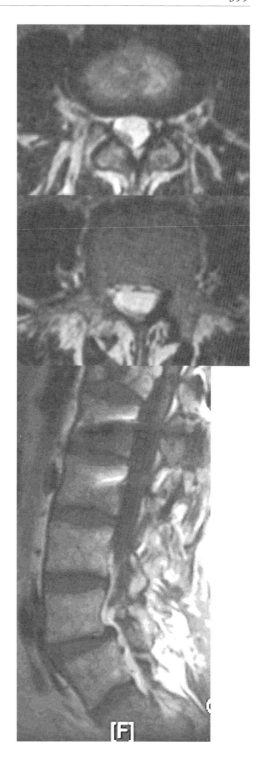